Dr. Kidd Guide to

MW01006586

Herbal Dog Care

Randy Kidd, D.V.M., Ph.D.

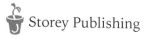
Storey Publishing

The mission of Storey Publishing is to serve our customers by
publishing practical information that encourages
personal independence in harmony with the environment.

Edited by Deborah Burns, Robin Catalano and Karen Levy
Cover design by Meredith Maker
Cover photograph of dog by Photodisc; cover photograph of garden by Giles
    Prett
Back cover illustration and animal illustrations by Rick Daskam
Herbal illustrations by Bobbi Angell, Kathy Bray, Sarah Brill, Beverly Duncan,
    Brigita Fuhrmann, Regina Hughes, Charles Joslin, Alison Kolesar, Susan
    Berry Langsten, Doug Paisley, and Elayne Sears
Text design and production by Susan Bernier and Jennifer Jepson Smith
Indexed by Susan Olason

Printed in the United States by Versa Press
10 9 8 7 6

Library of Congress Cataloging-in-Publication Data

Kidd, Randy, 1942–
    [Guide to herbal dog care]
    Dr. Kidd's guide to herbal dog care/Randy Kidd.
        p. cm.
    ISBN 978-1-58017-189-2 (pbk. : alk. paper)
    1. Dogs—Diseases—Alternative treatment. 2. Herbs—Therapeutic
use. 3. Herbals. 4. Holistic veterinary medicine. I. Title.
SF991 .K54 2000
636.7'08955—dc21   00-061874

Contents

Acknowledgments

Writers draw strength and inspiration from many sources, and I'd like to acknowledge three statements of belief that have formed the foundation of my approach to holistic veterinary medicine:

"In the beginning of all things, wisdom and knowledge were with the animals; for Tirawa, the One Above, did not speak directly to man. He sent certain animals to tell man that he showed himself through the beasts, and that from them, and from the stars and the sun and the moon, man should learn."
Chief Latakots-Lesa, Pawnee Tribe

"We believe that the domestic animals were sent here to accept the diseases of humans . . . and to show them how to heal these diseases."
Tis Mal Crow, Native American "Root Doctor"

"If there were no plants we would not be here. We breathe in what they breathe out. That is how we learn from them."
Keetoowah, Cherokee Teacher

I would also like to thank my hundreds of four-legged patients for their role as my personal teachers. My wife Sue, the matriarch of our family, has always been my strength, my way of staying rooted to the wellness that ultimately comes from our Earth Mother. Finally, I'd like to thank the family of folks at Storey Books for their editorial input and for having the faith that this book will help your pet's health, naturally.

part 1

Introducing Herbs

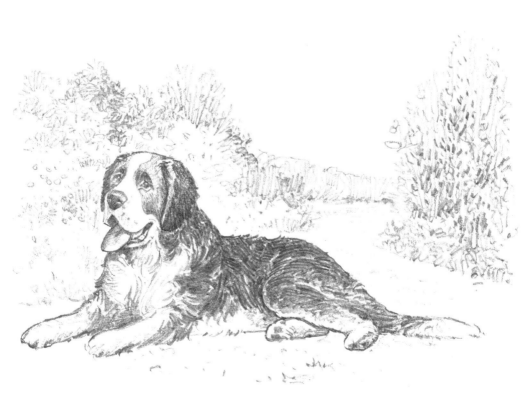

Introduction to Herbalism

Herbs have been an integral part of humankind's diet and pharmacy since we began roaming the earth. Some 5,000 years ago, the ancient Sumerians left written evidence of medicinal uses for plants such as laurel, caraway, and thyme. But long before the written word, caveman cultures left evidence of herbal use in their coprolites, or fossilized excrement. Herbalists have practiced their trade since the beginning of recorded history and in all parts of the world. Many herbs are mentioned in the Bible.

Typically, the plants of yore were used in unity with nature; their medicinal uses were based on humans' intuitive feel for their application along with observed results. Herbal use was often combined with practices such as shamanism, bleeding, fumigation, poulticing, rubbing, and urtication. In addition, most cultures had a ritualistic approach to planting and harvesting and to the collection of wild species.

Today, our culture so relies on Western medicines that we have lost our perspective on herbs. But herbs are used by more people worldwide than any other medicine. You probably don't have to go very far back in your own family history (perhaps to your grandmother or great-aunt) to discover an herbalist, someone who used the local "weeds" to cure all sorts of ailments.

Despite all this herbal history and lore, folks sometimes seem reluctant to use herbal medicines to help their pets. Concerned animal lovers have questions: Are the herbs safe to use? Which ones can I use for my dog? When should I use herbs, and are they ever more appropriate than the drugs of Western medicine? Should I use capsules, teas, tinctures, or topical preparations? How do I dose these treatments? And finally, are herbal medicines effective?

This book is designed to answer those questions. Herbs have been an integral part of my holistic veterinary practice for the past 10 years, and they have also been a part of my family's health care for several generations. Herbs are so safe and effective as helpers for other alternative medicines that I give almost every one of my patients an herbal prescription. And after years of use on hundreds of doggie patients — including my own dogs — I have found herbs so safe (when used correctly) that I am extremely comfortable prescribing them for all critters, even the most profoundly sick.

WHAT IS HOLISTIC MEDICINE?

I am a holistic veterinarian and have been for about 10 years now. I use a variety of "medicines" in my practice: herbs, acupuncture (Traditional Chinese Medicine), homeopathy, spinal and limb adjustments (chiropractic), nutrition and nutritional supplements, flower essences, shamanism, and more. Occasionally, I even resort to the Western or allopathic medicine I learned in veterinary school. I use what I think will be best for the patient at that particular time in his or her life cycle. And over the years I've found that, more often than not, the alternative medicines I choose *do* work.

Holistic medicine is much more than the "medicines" used. It is an approach to wellness that regards the patient as a whole organism, an organism that is intimately connected to its natural environment and whose health is tied to the health and well-being of the other organisms (including humans) around it.

St.-John's-wort

How Does Holistic Medicine Work?

Holistic medicine assumes that a diseased part of the organism is merely an expression of the fact that a lack of balance exists somewhere within the body. A holistic practitioner, when seeking a cure for any disease, aims to create a balance among all the body's organ systems.

To effect that cure, a holistic practitioner must be able to look at the patient from many different perspectives. Each of the medicines I use — herbal, homeopathic, Eastern, chiropractic, Western — has its own diagnostic and therapeutic methodology. And each of these methodologies is an independent system of its own, often complex and intricate in its approach and certainly highly refined by years of successful use by countless practitioners and patients.

As a holistic practitioner, then, I need to look at the patient from "many sides of the mountain."

Taking Responsibility for Health and the Planet

An aspect of holistic medicine that I feel is critical to the overall concept of "wholism" is that the medicine must be natural and must not deplete or pollute the environment.

Finally, and perhaps most important, I believe that holistic medicine — and especially the use of herbal remedies — is a prime way of empowering people to take charge of their pets' health . . . and their own. When using herbal medicines, you are the specialist. As an herbalist you realize that foods (and especially herbs) are medicine, and medicine is food, and you give Pet a boost with a daily dose of healthy herbs. Herbs are readily available over the counter for easy access. You don't need someone with a bunch of letters after her name to write a prescription just so you can use herbs; you can use herbs because you know they are safe and effective and because they work in a wide variety of situations, often affecting several organ systems at once.

You don't need a zillion bucks' worth of diagnostic and treatment machinery to support your healing methods, either. The herbs are there for you because that's their job: healing. And, perhaps best of all, you can grow healthy herbs in your very own backyard. While they are growing, you get the benefit of touching Mother Earth, and you have the opportunity to be in contact with and to smell healing herbs. After all, the largest organ of the body is the skin, and the most primitive organ is the nose. The healing qualities of many herbs are readily absorbed through the skin, and aromatherapy is an age-old healing method.

MY BEGINNINGS AS A PRACTICING HERBALIST

While my family has made extensive use of herbs seemingly forever, my dog Rufus finally convinced me to use them in my practice. (Remember, like all my veterinary colleagues, my previous training was exclusively Western-medicine oriented.)

Rufus: My First Case Study

Just about the time I started studying alternative medicines, Rufus, a totally lovable golden retriever with the usual complement of three brain cells, got a "hot spot" on his forearm. Hot spots are skin irritations of unknown cause; they usually begin as small, itchy areas that the animal may lick and bite until the spots are raw and bleeding. In Western medicine, hot spots are commonly treated with cortisone ointment, an anti-inflammatory.

I gave Rufus the best of Western medicine, slathering on the cortisone ointment. His hot spot went away almost immediately. But it returned in a few months — redder, angrier, and itchier. So I went to the bigger "guns" of Western medicine: oral cortisone pills, given in addition to the topical ointment.

The hot spot disappeared, this time after 3 or 4 days, only to return again in a few months. The spot was redder yet; much larger; and, according to Rufus, so itchy that it was nearly impossible to bear. I gave him another dose of cortisone, this time in ointment, injectable, and follow-up pill form.

The hot spot again disappeared, this time after a week or so. But in a few weeks it came back with a vengeance, and Rufus let us know he was miserable, day and night. Well, you get the picture. Western medicines in general, and cortisone products in particular, typically work by palliating diseases — making patients feel better for short periods of time without really curing them.

Calendula

Finding Success with Herbs

Deep into my alternative medicine studies, I decided to apply what I'd learned to Rufus. (Much like the shoemaker's daughter who never has shoes, most veterinarian's pets are the last to get treated.) From the few herbal books I had at the time, I learned that calendula is a good herb for healing reddened, raw skin lesions. Sue, my wife, had some calendula growing in the garden, so we picked it, steeped it into a mild tea, and spritzed it on Rufus's ever-growing hot spot.

"Ahhh." I could almost hear Rufus's sigh of relief as he settled down, quit scratching, and relaxed for the first time in days. In a few hours the itch recurred, so we applied another spritz. Immediate relief. After four or five treatments throughout that first day, Rufus experienced no itching, and he had a good night's sleep for the first time in weeks. Then, amazingly, the very next morning I could see evidence of wound healing around the edges of the hot spot — nice white, clean tissue growth.

Well, after a few days of herbal spritz, Rufus's hot spot completely disappeared, and it has never returned. I was really happy for Rufus (and for us, since we could now sleep in peace), but I wondered why I didn't learn about calendula or any of the other herbs in veterinary school. But that's another story.

After watching Rufus's results, I was hooked. I began using herbs extensively from that day on, recommending them for all my patients.

HOW TO USE THIS BOOK

My guide to herbal dog care is designed to make it easy for you to begin using herbs on your pooch right away. Please read the first section before you jump into the chapters on organ systems and the herbal repertory.

Chapters 4 and 5 are designed to help you understand the how-tos of herb use. There's nothing difficult about it; herbal medicine is not rocket science. I am a veterinarian/herbalist who thinks that herbal medicine is the most empowering of the alternative medicines because herbs are meant to be used by everyone, including your dog. *You* can choose to create a healthy internal and external environment by growing and feeding healthy herbs to your family of animals. *You* can choose to use herbs because they are safe and effective. And, as you use herbs, *you* can learn about your own environment and the place that herbs have in it.

Start using herbs today. Sprinkle a sample of a tonic herb atop Rover's food. If he doesn't like that tonic, try another. Keep trying until you find the herbs he likes. Make a light herbal tea and pour it over his food, or try adding some to his water.

To keep your dog healthy, use herbs on a daily basis. If you should ever need them, you'll have much better luck getting a sick pooch to agree to herbal medicines if she has been acclimated to them over the years.

Then, if your dog ever comes down with the "sicks," all you need is a diagnosis from your "regular" veterinarian to tell you which organ system is affected or which problem your dog has. With the diagnosis in hand, go to the chapter that lists the herbs for that organ system, and use the plants as directed. It couldn't be simpler.

Now, there is a minor rub to all this: Whenever you choose to use herbal medicine — or any other alternative medicine, for that matter — you likely won't get much *(any)* help from your conventional vet. Most vets are simply not trained in holistic health. But holistic veterinarians are now located in all parts of the country (see Resources), and many of them are available for either office or phone consultations. In any emergency, of course, you should contact your regular vet — or a local emergency veterinary clinic, if one is available in your area.

FOR MORE INFORMATION

For those of you who want to continue your herbal studies, or for those who want to have some more fun with herbs, check out our two Web sites: www.HonoringTheAnimals.com and www.HookedOnHerbs.com.

10 Steps to Holistic Health Care for Dogs

As I've mentioned, holistic practice involves much more than any one medicine. So, early on in my holistic practice, I developed a protocol that has helped me think in terms of wholism — an integrated approach to creating whole-body-mind-heart-spirit health for Pet (and for Pet's people). I know many holistic practitioners who refer to this holistic balance simply as body-mind-spirit (or body-mind-soul). But I add the heart because I've always thought of the heart as an internal organ AND a source of energy, while I see the spirit as more outwardly oriented — coming from some unknown source but dramatically affecting all internal organs. This heart-spirit split may be merely semantics, but it gives me the opportunity to describe and work with problems such as an animal's "broken heart" over the loss of a family member or an animal's heartfelt passion to be with his humans. (Interestingly, Traditional Chinese Medicine has a term, *Shen*, that is identified as "spirit," or the substance unique to human life. Shen resides in the heart, along with what the Chinese view as the mind.) In addition, my protocol has helped me see where the herbs fit (or at least where *I* think they fit) in an overall approach to wellness.

For my protocol I use a highly scientific model: one of those bathtub toys made for kids. (My idea for using the toy came as I watched one of our grandkids splash in the tub — what could be more healthy than watching kids or pets have fun?) This protocol forces us to be aware of the holistic perspective of wellness. It also helps us apply in proper sequence the healing methods we ultimately select. And from its format, we can learn to think about *all* aspects of health in a logical, sequential manner.

DR. KIDD'S HOLISTIC PROTOCOL FOR HEALTH: AS ONE WITH NATURE

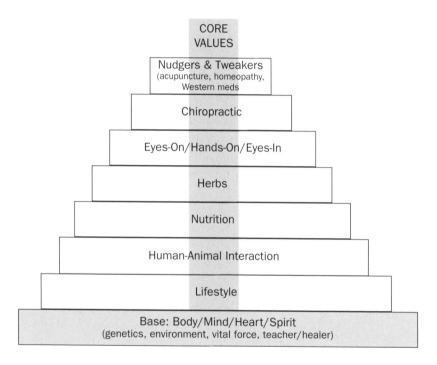

CORE VALUES

Nudgers & Tweakers (acupuncture, homeopathy, Western meds

Chiropractic

Eyes-On/Hands-On/Eyes-In

Herbs

Nutrition

Human-Animal Interaction

Lifestyle

Base: Body/Mind/Heart/Spirit (genetics, environment, vital force, teacher/healer)

HOW TO INTERPRET THE MODEL

This protocol is based on a direct connection with Mother Earth, creating a basis for holistic health that relies on living *naturally*. In addition, any holistic approach to health will create a natural balance of body, mind, heart, and spirit.

The Foundation: As One with Nature

I think it helps to visualize this model as resting on a healthy Mother Earth and seeking natural ways to evaluate and perpetuate health. Then, envision an application of the protocol that includes a natural way to balance all aspects of body, mind, heart, and spirit. Finally, think in terms of the animal being able to heal itself by working with its own innate powers. This, then, is the first and perhaps most important step in the protocol — realizing that everything we do for ourselves and for our animals is based on the premise that we are nature, that we are all one with nature. The realization of our interconnectedness with nature will ultimately make us and our pets whole and healthy.

Just as you would begin with the base when building anything with structural integrity, you must establish a firm foundation for holistic health. Next, look closely at each of the rings, proceeding from the larger rings at the bottom to the smaller rings at the top. The larger the ring, the greater the required emphasis on that area of health.

Also, remember that as we proceed from the bottom to the top of the model, our ability to tweak the patient's vital force *(chi)* toward wellness is progressively stronger — as are our chances to harm the patient if our method is not applied properly. This means that we should not use any of the potent medicines, including homeopathy, chiropractic, and acupuncture, unless we have the knowledge base that comes from adequate training in the method.

The Base

The base, or foundation, of our model is made up of several factors. All of these factors must be present for optimum health.

Genetics. The basis of any wellness program is a genetic foundation that produces immune-competent and socially adaptable animals. Healthy animals also need a body structure that is adapted to the type of work they are asked to do and a biomechanical integrity that is conducive to a balanced flow of inner vitality. For example, consider the low-slung dachshund, bred to be a hunting dog that could easily enter small burrows to flush out prey. Fine and dandy, but when we ask that body type to jump over hurdles (as we may do in agility drills) or run up and down stairs, we put undue stress on the muscles, tendons, and joints of the lower back and shoulders. Now compare the dachshund to the greyhound, which has the perfect body type for speed running. But we wouldn't expect the greyhound to crawl into tiny spaces without putting stress on its joints and tendons.

Environment. All animals (including humans) have the right to live in a pollution-free, stress-free, toxin-free environment — an outer environment that allows the animal to meet its natural needs as much as possible.

Vital force. For whole-body-mind-heart-spirit wellness, the vital force (or chi, or innateness, or spirit, or orgone, or whatever else you might want to call it) must be able to grow to its capacity. I've found herbs, especially when used with the energetic medicines of homeopathy and acupuncture, to be vital in this area.

Animals as teachers and healers. The essence of our association with animals is to love and honor them as teachers — our very best models for natural, holistic health.

The Lower Rings

Each of the rings that sit atop the base of our model corresponds to a different aspect of holistic health care.

Lifestyle. Every lifestyle choice a person or family makes has the potential to affect the overall health of the animals in the home. Smoking not only harms the smoker but also damages her dog's lungs through secondary exposure to smoke. But when a family eats a wholesome, organic, balanced diet, the dog has the advantage of getting healthy table scraps. And when the family takes the dog for a daily walk, all of the walkers benefit from the exercise.

Human-animal interaction. All animals crave interaction with other living beings. Research shows that merely touching an animal lowers a person's heart rate. Human conversations even become quieter in the presence of animals. And simply watching animals — a fish in an aquarium is enough — calms the observers and lowers their blood pressure. It's clear that the animals, too, need the benefit of touch, from other animals and from humans. The impressive part of human-animal interactions is that they work so well as a positive feedback system: The more we

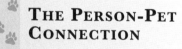

THE PERSON-PET CONNECTION

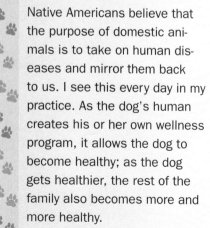

Native Americans believe that the purpose of domestic animals is to take on human diseases and mirror them back to us. I see this every day in my practice. As the dog's human creates his or her own wellness program, it allows the dog to become healthy; as the dog gets healthier, the rest of the family also becomes more and more healthy.

touch and rub and hug, the more each of us benefits. The healthier we become, the healthier our pets are, too.

Nutrition. The best food for all animals (including humans) is organic and natural. The worst is derived from diseased meat scraps, grains produced with heavy doses of herbicides and pesticides, highly cooked foods, and feed laden with artificial preservatives or flavorings. If you provide the best-quality nutrients available, 90 percent of your dog's health problems will miraculously disappear. Remember that herbs are also healthy foods.

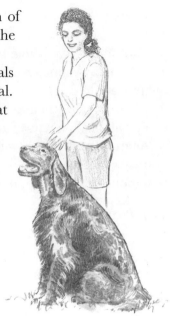

Regular interaction with your dog is integral to her general health and well-being.

The Middle Rings

Building on the base and the lower rings, the middle rings can be viewed as important supplemental health-care methods.

Herbs. Herbs can provide a full spectrum of impact on the vital force. Many herbs can be used as vitamin- and immune-enhancing supplements, some are mild tonics or stimulants for numerous organ systems, and others are used as acute treatments. Although I've found some herbs to be extremely effective as therapeutic medicinals, I generally consider them to be supportive for other health modalities. Typically the effects of herbs are very subtle, and it takes time (often 30 to 90 days) before we see positive results.

Hands-On, Eyes-In, Eyes-On. A vital link from your heart to your dog's heart is through your hands and through the positive images you produce of your dog's continuing health. Easy-to-learn massage techniques (hands-on) will help transfer your innate healing powers to your dog, and the use of positive imagery (eyes-in) will enhance any healthy method used for you or your dog. Another key to a holistic health program is to properly evaluate your dog's ongoing condition. Good observational skills (eyes-on) and the maintenance of a detailed journal are invaluable aids while you are helping Pet become and remain healthy.

Chiropractic. Many types of musculoskeletal pain or gait abnormalities can be eased with chiropractic care, and routine adjustments may be helpful for the athletic animal or human. In addition, a musculoskeletal system with a "kink" in it will not allow the vital force to flow freely. Often, a simple chiropractic adjustment frees the animal's innate ability to balance and heal itself.

Using Flower Essences

Flower essences, also known as Bach Flower Remedies, are herbal products that have a dramatic effect on an animal's mental, psychic, or spiritual condition. I often combine them with other modalities as a further boost to an animal's whole wellness program. You can purchase flower essences at natural food stores and through mail-order suppliers (see Resources).

The Upper Rings: Nudgers and Tweakers

As you can see in the illustration on page 9, the top ring — the nudgers and tweakers — is the smallest ring. Nudgers and tweakers have their place in health care, but for long-term and in-depth holistic health, they are the least important of all the health methods.

Western medicine. Since it is the medicine most healing practitioners in the United States learn in school, Western, or allopathic, medicine is the predominant medicine practiced in the United States. While all holistic practitioners are very aware of allopathic medicine's limitations, some allopathic applications have a place in any holistic practice. For example, allopathic medicine works very well for treating acute bacterial infections and traumatic injuries.

Acupuncture. Technically, acupuncture is only a portion of Traditional Chinese Medicine (TCM). True TCM also includes the use of Chinese herbs, lifestyle changes, chi mind/body exercises, and proper nutrition. Most practitioners in the United States, however, use acupuncture as the major part of TCM.

By selectively placing acupuncture needles along the naturally occurring meridians (lines of chi flow that were mapped out thou-

sands of years ago) of
an animal whose chi
is not balanced,
the practitioner
achieves a healthy flow
of chi that ultimately balances the animal's inner and
outer wellness. Although TCM has
been used for nearly all ailments in
almost all species, it has proved to be

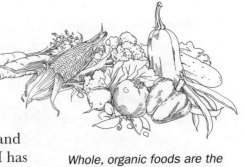

*Whole, organic foods are the
foundation of a healthy diet.*

especially helpful in animals (human and nonhuman) with painful
musculoskeletal diseases.

Homeopathy. Homeopathy uses extremely diluted, natural substances (remedies) — from animal, vegetable, and mineral sources
— that enable an animal's vital force to expand to its full capacity,
eliminating the potential for impending diseases. The basis for
homeopathy is that "like cures like," and healing remedies are
selected according to the properties they have demonstrated in
trials conducted on healthy people and animals. Homeopathic
remedies have proved effective in all sorts of diseases, including
metabolic and musculoskeletal conditions.

Core Values

The central part of the model, the part that holds it all together,
is what I call core values. Everyone has a set of core values that
they believe in. A person's spiritual belief system is one example of
a core value, and this value carries with it a tremendous capacity
for healing. Whatever your spiritual preference, prayer is highly
recommended — and has proved to be effective — as a healing
method for the entire family.

Wrapping It Up

So there you have the protocol I've found tremendously helpful
in trying to decide on the best holistic method for long-term and in-
depth healing in an animal patient. Everything is based on a natural approach — the entire protocol rests on Mother Earth, the
basic premise of As One with Nature.

Herbs comprise the middle ring. In my mind, this is the perfect
place for them because they are central in any healing program.

Herbal medicine can be utilized throughout the entire spectrum of healing: Herbs are nutritious, balancing to organ systems (or entire organisms), stimulating, and energetically healing.

When to Use Nudgers and Tweakers

I consider all the powerful medicines I use — Western medicine, acupuncture (TCM), and homeopathy — as mere nudgers and tweakers because that's exactly how I see them work clinically. Any of these medicines has the capacity to nudge or tweak your dog into a healthier state of balance — at least temporarily.

However, for long-term wellness, I've found that it is absolutely essential to establish a firm foundation of health (as per my holistic protocol). Otherwise, our "cures" are typically short term and the disease returns — either in its original form or in another, often worse, chronic form of disease.

The major mistake of modern medicine, as I see it, is that it has flipped the protocol's pyramid and uses as its primary treatments the top, or smallest of the rings: the nudgers and tweakers. With this flip-flop, we have created a medicine without foundation, a medicine that has almost no structural integrity — a medicine that may work for the short term but does not create long-lasting health.

Even worse, most of today's "medicine folk" have removed from their thinking the central peg, the core or spiritual values of the protocol's pyramid. Without the core value of spirituality, the pyramid has even less stability.

With rare exceptions, the nudger and tweaker medicines I use are acupuncture and homeopathy. I have chosen these medicines because they are highly effective (more so than most of the Western medicines I used years ago); they are based on the way nature works; and when used properly, they help restore my patients to a long-term balance of body, mind, heart, and spirit.

Using Herbs
for Health

From my perspective as a holistic practitioner, herbs offer the best of all worlds. They have a full spectrum of activity, from mildly nutritional to powerfully medicinal. With this broad activity, herbal medicine gives us the opportunity to choose the plants that will most likely help our patient.

Herbs are not drugs. For those of us with an allopathic background, this concept can be extremely difficult to grasp. But if we are to use herbs successfully on our dogs, it is absolutely essential that we understand this basic difference between drugs and herbs.

An herb is *not* one single bioactive chemical that a practitioner uses specifically to alter a biochemical process that has gone awry. Instead, each and every herb contains dozens of bioactive chemicals. As we'll see later, this potpourri of bioactive chemicals has advantages and drawbacks. Generally, herbs:

- **Are nutritious.** They add proteins, carbohydrates, vitamins, minerals, and other important nutrients (such as antioxidants) to the diet.
- **Add spice.** As well as being nutritious, and in many cases medicinal, culinary herbs add taste to foods. Spices not only enhance the flavor but also improve digestion by activating digestive juices and enzymes. Often just the odor of a spice will kick the digestive system into full gear.

- **Are tonic.** Many herbs have a tonic effect on the body, help-ing maintain the balance of the body's organ systems. A tonic herb will either stimulate or relax its target systems, depending on what is needed. (See page 21 for more information.)
- **Have specific medicinal uses.** Herbs used as medicine have a specific activity on one or several organ systems. For instance, catnip is used to relax the nervous system, and it also has the ability to help clear up stomach upsets, such as colic, dyspep-sia, and flatulence. Or herbs may be used to create a general-ized physiological effect — sweating, for example.

CAUTION

Herbs can be beneficial, but if they are used incorrectly they may be toxic or even lethal. However, the risk of adverse side effects and death is far less when using herbs than when using Western medi-cine's drugs. Most of the herbal reactions seen are idiosyncratic, which means that they occur only in the rare individual who has a personal allergy to something in the herb. The adverse reaction is generally mild, and the reaction almost always stops when use of the herb is discontinued. Signs of adverse reactions are those you'd expect with any allergy: runny eyes and nose, sneezing, itching (any-where on the body), swelling, and possibly diarrhea or vomiting.

The potential for adverse reactions is increased when we take a single part of the plant (as in allopathic medicine) and use it in con-centrations higher than those found in nature. But when we use an herb as a whole plant and not an extracted "active ingredient," we have almost no problems with adverse reactions.

It is estimated that 10,000 deaths a year are caused by allopathic drugs. Some experts even say that this number is two or three times too low. If you added up all the deaths from herbal use, you *might* come up with 100 over a 10-year period. You do the math.

- **Can have primary or secondary uses.** An example of a primary herb is echinacea, which balances the immune system. Echinacea has a specific action that increases lymphocyte production and activity when needed and decreases lymphocyte production when enough lymphocytes are already present. Secondary herbs have activity associated with the organ system of concern but do not necessarily directly affect it. For example, dandelion root acts as a diuretic, helping cleanse and nourish the urinary system. But I also often include it as a secondary herb for cardiac patients because many animals with heart problems have a difficult time eliminating fluids.
- **Can be contraindicated.** Some herbs should not be used during specific times in the life cycle, such as pregnancy. These herbs are toxic enough that indiscriminate and prolonged use can lead to illness or even death. In addition, a few plants can be lethal, even in small, one-time doses. Proper disease diagnosis, plant identification, and dosage are absolutely necessary.

DIAGNOSING AND PRESCRIBING

Correct diagnosis is essential in order to apply any medicine properly, and herbal medicine is no exception. However, each medical modality has its own diagnostic specifics. Chinese medicine, for example, makes extensive use of tongue and pulse diagnosis. Classical homeopathy uses the totality of symptoms (without much regard to *why* the symptoms occur), while chiropractic uses joint flexibility and function as its primary diagnostic aids.

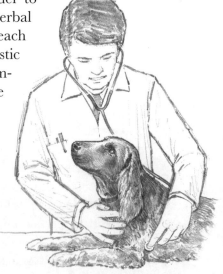

In herbal medicine, my primary interest is to determine which organ system is "out of whack" and needs to be returned to normal. Then, after I've determined the herbs specific for the affected organ system, I try to select herbs that will help other

Always consult a qualified veterinarian before starting a treatment program.

body systems that are also stressed by the dog's condition. In my practice, I follow a four-step process for diagnosing and prescribing.

Step 1: A Good Western Medicine Diagnosis

We need to know which organ system is compromised; we do not necessarily need to know the precise cause of the disease (though that can be helpful). Western medicine has excellent diagnostic tools for determining when an organ system is not normal; complete blood counts (CBCs), urinalysis, blood chemistries, X rays, magnetic resonance imaging (MRI), or ultrasound diagnosis might be indicated.

Let's say that these tests indicate a dysfunctional urinary tract. In that case you would go to chapter 21 and select from among the herbs that are listed as primary for the urinary system.

Step 2: Look for Outside Factors

Is this condition infectious or noninfectious? Are we dealing with excessive or abnormal cellular growth (cancer) or decreased cellular function (possibly from changes associated with old age)? Is it an immune problem? If so, is something attacking the immune system from outside or is your dog's body attacking his own immune system from the inside? Are outside toxins a possibility or is Fido's body simply unable to eliminate his daily production of internal waste products?

From the answers to these questions, we would have information with which to select secondary herbs to help restore the whole body to normal. If, to continue our above example, the urinary problem is infectious (caused by bacteria or viruses), we would want to prescribe herbs with antibiotic potential as well as herbs to enhance the immune system in general.

Step 3: Evaluate Other Factors

Are there any other factors that may be implicated in the whole disease — factors that we can help alleviate with herbs? For example, in nearly any disease, your dog will need to eliminate toxic products generated as a result of tissue inflammation, loss of normal function, or infection. The body's primary organ for toxin elimination is the liver, so most of my herbal prescriptions include liver-helper herbs.

Step 4: Choose Facilitators

Are there any herbs that may facilitate the transport or delivery of other herbs to target organs? Cayenne, for example, acts to improve circulation in general, which helps move bioactive chemicals from herbs into areas where they are needed.

INCLUDING TONICS IN HEALTH CARE

According to Daniel P. Mowery, Ph.D., in *Herbal Tonic Therapies* (Keats Publishing, 1993), a tonic herb is any substance that balances the biochemical and physiological events that comprise body systems. Scientists use the word *homeostasis* to describe this balance; *normality* and *equilibrium* are other frequently used terms for the same purpose. Keep in mind that a tonic does not just stimulate a body system; it acts to move the body back to an optimum state — stimulating or strengthening when necessary, or depressing, lowering, or relaxing when those actions are appropriate.

True tonic herbs also:

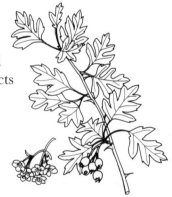

- Must be free of side effects
- Must have few or no contraindications
- Should be able to be consumed in small amounts daily without adverse side effects (including addiction and tolerance)
- May exhibit bidirectional characteristics (see the box on page 21)

A true tonic herb is recognized as such only after centuries of use by countless practitioners and patients.

Hawthorn

SAFETY AND EFFICACY: SYNERGY AND BIDIRECTIONALITY

All medical practitioners judge the medicines they use by two specific criteria: safety and efficacy. Is the medicine reasonably safe to use on the majority of my patients? Can I expect positive results (good efficacy) most of the time I use the medicine? Herbs fit the bill for both of these criteria.

Understanding Synergy

As we've already noted, every herbal plant contains a potpourri of bioactive chemicals. Many of these individual chemicals work together within your dog's body synergistically, in a combined action. This means the total reaction of the plant's bioactive parts can be much more than the sum of each of its component parts.

When you give your dog a whole herb, the synergy of all its parts will enhance its overall efficacy. But if you give Spot a pill that is a plant extract and contains only one of the plant's bioactive

---

My Favorite Tonics

Here are some tonics I use in my veterinary practice (see The Herbal Repertory for specifics on most of the plants and the parts used).

- **Immune system:** Echinacea, ginseng, astragalus *(Astragalus membranaceous)*, licorice
- **Cardiovascular system:** Hawthorn, one of the "seaweeds" (kelp or bladderwack, for example), turmeric, mother-wort, Siberian ginseng *(Eleutherococcus senticosus)*, valerian
- **Nervous system:** Valerian, ginkgo *(Ginkgo biloba)*, hop *(Humulus lupulus)*, peppermint *(Mentha x piperita)*, chamomile, Siberian ginseng *(Eleutherococcus senticosus)*, lemon balm *(Melissa officinalis)*
- **Digestive system:** Milk thistle, artichoke *(Cynara scolymus)*, dandelion, ginger, turmeric
- **Musculoskeletal system:** Alfalfa *(Medicago sativa)*, devil's claw *(Harpagophytum procumbens)*, yarrow, saw palmetto, wild yam *(Dioscorea villosa)*, echinacea, licorice, sarsaparilla
- **Female reproductive system:** Dong quai, ginger, black haw *(Viburnum prunifolium)*, cramp bark *(Viburnum spp.)*, valerian, raspberry *(Rubus idaeus)*, licorice, black cohosh, chaste tree *(Vitex agnus-castus)*
- **Male reproductive system:** Pygeum *(Pygeum africanum)*, pumpkin *(Cucurbita pepo)*, sarsaparilla, saw palmetto *(Serenoa repens)*, Siberian ginseng *(Eleutherococcus senticosus)*

ingredients, then Spot receives the effects of only that one active ingredient. This is not always bad, since we may want to produce a very specific action on the body. But in general, herbs are better used in toto; when used whole, all of the herb's bioactive ingredients work in synergy to positively affect your dog's entire body.

The Benefits of Bidirectionality

Bidirectionality means that a plant, through its many individual components, may direct its actions to one part or system of the body when needed but may have the opposite action if that is needed. Daniel Mowery refers to this concept as "specific hunger": the ability of animals and humans to select from a menu of foods containing nutrients the body is lacking at the time, thus restoring or maintaining homeostasis. Bidirectionality enhances herbal safety because the herbs help the body return to a balanced state. In addition, because one herb can be used for many different diseases, efficacy is increased.

Ginseng, for instance, contains two bioactive ingredients: Rb ginsenosides and Rg ginsenosides. Each ingredient has an opposing action on blood pressure. Rb ginsenosides lower blood pressure; Rg ginsenosides raise it. These opposing actions help balance blood pressure. Ginseng also contains components that raise blood sugar and others that lower blood sugar. Hawthorn berries, like ginseng, tend to help normalize both high and low blood pressure.

To give another example, echinacea, with its ability to act in two opposing directions, brings almost every aspect of immune function under control. If your dog has a lower than normal white cell count, echinacea acts to increase production of white cells in the bone marrow. But if your dog's white cell count is high, echinacea decelerates production of those cells.

Echinacea

Note that if we use a one-ingredient extract of a bidirectional herb, it will *not* have a bidirectional effect.

Echinacea and Immunity

In addition to having a bidirectional effect on white cell production, echinacea stabilizes the cell membrane of the histamine-containing mast cell in animals that have symptoms from allergies. This is contrary to most immune-enhancers, which sensitize the animal that has allergies.

Have Herbs Been Scientifically Proved to Work?

The answer to this question is an emphatic yes, but . . .

Science, good science, is nothing more — and nothing less — than the unbiased observation of phenomena. Sounds simple enough, but it isn't. If it were simple, we would be able to say that many of the uses of medicinal herbs have been scientifically validated. After all, millions of users over eons should provide adequate testimony.

Furthermore, many of the medicinal uses of herbs have been validated through the most rigorous scientific testing. This testing uses validation studies in which randomly selected subjects are treated with either a placebo or an herb. The studies are "double blind," so neither the patient nor the doctor knows who receives the placebo and who receives the herb. Some herbs have been tested on animals, while others have been tested on humans. Still other tests have been done on both animal and human subjects.

But chances are your veterinarian or physician has never seen those studies. Many of the tests have been conducted overseas and, for some reason, the community of healers in the United States tends to disregard anything that is not from within its own boundaries. What's more, many of the scientifically valid studies performed in the United States never reach the journals your veterinarian (or physician) reads; those journals are heavily funded by commercial pharmaceutical companies. As you can guess, those companies aren't wild about you replacing their expensive drugs with "weeds" from your own backyard. So good scientific studies on herbal care for dogs are not always easy to find.

And the problems run even deeper than that. Our reductionist model of medicine tries to boil down a disease to its smallest biochemical reason and then attempts to apply a chemical to "attack and cure" the problem. This mentality is only natural for scientists (and even some herbalists), who like to think that there is one bioactive chemical hidden within an herb or a drug that will cure a specific disease. But we've already seen that this is not true for herbs, because they have a veritable plethora of bioactive ingredients that act both synergistically and bidirectionally.

What is the concerned dog companion to do? Read on for some suggestions.

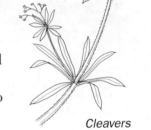
Cleavers

Whole Plants vs. Extracts

When used in whole rather than extracted form, herbs are incredibly safe medicines. Well-known tonic herbs produce almost no adverse reactions. Millions of users throughout history can't all be wrong.

But whenever we alter the original whole-plant package, we can create trouble for our dogs. Since extracts do not contain an herb's protective bidirectional ingredients, the one biochemical that has been extracted may be concentrated to a toxic level. Remember: Part of an herb's protective mechanism is that vast amounts of any one chemical are not usually concentrated in the herb's leaves, roots, or flowers.

On the other hand, because most herbs lack huge concentrations of a specific bioactive substance, they often create a mild medicinal reaction in patients. Herbs usually act in subtle ways, and it may be weeks to months before you'll see any reaction in your dog. For my patients, especially for those with chronic conditions, I appreciate this slow and subtle reaction; "slow and easy" perfectly complements my other, specific medicines.

Find a Reputable Practitioner

The first step in successful herbal treatment is to find an herbalist or a holistic practitioner you can trust (see Resources for more information). Your trustworthy practitioner should have a good scientific background along with the horse sense to apply and then evaluate herbal medicines in clinical situations. Let the practitioner be the one to evaluate the scientific validity of claims made about an herb, as well as the clinical applications of that herb.

Choose Your Herbs Wisely

Use herbs that have been proved to be safe and effective over generations of use by multitudes of folks. Part 3 gives you a good base of herbs from which to choose. Whenever possible, use the tonic herbs. Avoid what I call the designer herbs — those plants that are the current media darlings, such as yucca, devil's claw, and chapparal — until they have been around long enough to be properly evaluated in a clinical and scientific environment.

ARE DOUBLE-BLIND STUDIES REALLY THE ANSWER?

Even though double-blind studies really do not remove examiner bias, our scientists continue to insist on the double-blind study as their gold standard for testing. But not all herbs have been scientifically validated, and some of the most popular ones — such as kava kava, ginkgo, and ma huang — have not even withstood the scrutiny of time and trial. Because scientists insist on double-blind studies, they tend to ignore the practical, at-home trials that have been conducted for centuries by millions of people around the world. But even the most controlled scientific study cannot remove all of the outside factors that affect results, so we need to think in terms of whether a treatment is making the patient feel better. The simplest way to determine effectiveness is to ask yourself how bad your dog was doing before treatment. Then ask how well he is doing after treatment. If there is improvement, the treatment is working effectively. If none, perhaps not. If he's getting worse, certainly not. In this way, you and your holistic vet can decide on the best course of treatment.

TODAY'S MOST POPULAR OR "DESIGNER" HERBS

Almost every month a blitz of media reports will ballyhoo a particular herb as God's gift for some disease or another, often citing several ecstatic users and their remarkable recoveries. Blah blah blah. Read magazines and newspapers from the past and you'll find adoring articles extolling the virtues of herbs such as kava kava, St.-John's-wort, ginkgo, gotu kola, ma huang, chaparral, devil's claw, and yucca. The problem with these "designer" herbs is *not* that they are ineffective; many of them work well . . . when used correctly. The problem is that they can almost certainly NOT cure everything the media say they can. I tell folks: ALL medicines work . . . on some patients, some of the time. The key is to find the medicine that will work the best for *your individual* dog. I warn them not to get confused by the hyperbolic claims of the media and not to expect miracles from the herbs in today's news reports. Then I tell them to use the herbs as they were meant to be used — expecting slow and subtle results that create in-depth, long-term healing.

Become a Smart Consumer

Do not rely on media reports or on the stockperson in the health food or pet store for accurate information. Instead, refer to Resources in this book for good herbal magazines and become knowledgeable in general about herbs and their specific uses. After you complete your research, use the herbs for your dog's — and for your — health. Practical application is the very best way to educate and empower yourself.

And if you feel you must have scientific validation for a particular herb, remember to evaluate the studies that have used the *whole* herb, not an extracted biochemical. Results that apply to one biochemical almost never apply to the whole herb.

*Y*ou'd be surprised how many of my clients bring me an herb sold to them by a store clerk who has told them it would be good for their dog's problem. You'd probably not be surprised if I tell you that, nine times out of ten, the herb does not apply.

Learning about Herbs

At first glance, learning about herbs may seem an almost impossible task. There are, after all, thousands of herbs, and the medicinal aspects of herbology come packaged with foreign-sounding terminology and treatments. What's more, it often seems that each and every herb has dozens of practical, medicinal uses. Whew!

TIPS FOR YOUR HERBAL EDUCATION

Well, buck up, matey. You can make learning about herbs much easier on yourself by following a few practical tips. In fact, becoming acquainted with herbs can be the most enjoyable task you've ever undertaken. This chapter will tell you how to go about it.

Keep It Simple

Sure, there are several thousand medicinal herbs. So what? Do you need to know everything about all of them? Absolutely not! In fact, many traditional herbalists of the past used only 10 or 12 herbs in their entire practice. In a typical year I might use 30 or 40 herbs on a routine basis, with only a few more that I've added to help a rare patient — often after I've looked up and studied the seldom used herb, just for the patient's special needs.

Follow Your Interests

Herbs are truly the most fascinating study I've ever undertaken. Their medicinal actions in animals are most interesting. But so, too, are some of the folktales that involve herbs, their appearances in literature and visual art, their historical uses in various cultures, and their mythical and magical properties. Whatever your special interests and fascinations are, use them to make your herbal learning curve less steep. Remember that whenever we can attach a personal reason to our studies, the topic becomes much easier to learn.

Get to Know the Organ Systems

Perhaps you have a particular need to know about herbs. Maybe your dog has a heart condition, for example. Many herbs are heart helpful, and you could spend the next several months studying these herbs in general and how they affect the heart specifically. From this study you could decide which herbs would be best for Pooch's condition.

Join the Herb-of-the-Month Club

Nothing will drive learning better than a vital personal need to know. But if your family is free of diseases at the present, be happy and subscribe to the Herb-of-the-Month Club. Pick an herb — any herb — and take a month to study it. (Okay, you might be smarter than the rest of us, and you might be able to study two or three herbs every month, but be sure you do not bite off more herb than you can chew.) The secret is to really learn about one herb at a time.

Learn the herb's Latin name (see the box on page 30), where it grows and what it looks like, what parts are used medicinally, its general actions on

The Many Uses of Mullein

I began my herbal studies with mullein *(Verbascum thapsus)*. Over the years, whenever I've come across any new information pertaining to mullein, I've added it to my personal "Book of Mullein Lore," which now contains several dozen pages. Mullein has taken me down roads of learning I've never been on before and probably never would have traveled had it not been for this fascinating herb.

For example, did you know that the "moly" Mercury gave Ulysses to use as a charm against Circe's enchantments was mullein? Well, I didn't, but this bit of information encouraged me to read *The Odyssey* for the first time — which in turn began my fascination with the classics.

If you like historical trivia, you'll be interested to know that mullein was called the herb of love or herbe of protection in medieval times. In the seventh century, the herb was so important it was named herbe de St. Fiacre, after the Irish saint who became the patron saint of gardeners.

Mullein has long been thought to have both evil and good properties. One of its common names, hag's taper, refers to its supposed use as a transportation aid for witches in the days before broomsticks. Christian lore places mullein, or Heaven's Blaze, under Mary's protection, as per the old saying "Our dear Lady travels the land, carrying Heaven's Blaze in her hand."

We can also learn more about an herb from its historical uses. Roman ladies used mullein flowers to dye their hair blond, and Mormon women rubbed the rough leaves on their cheeks to create a red flush. Native Americans have used mullein seeds to paralyze fish (much like today's chemical rotenone), making them easy to gather as they float on a pond's surface.

Mullein is often thought of as a "protector plant." In olden days people hung mullein leaves in their homes to keep away negativity, and they stuffed the herb into pillows to guard against nightmares. Even today, European farmers refer to mullein as weathercandles, and they grow it close to their homes and outbuildings to keep lightning away.

body systems, and any contraindications for usage. Then learn tidbits about the herb that will connect it to your special interests (see "Follow Your Interests" on page 28) — like its folklore, magical uses, special medicinal uses for female or male systems, and so on.

By studying just one herb a month, in a few short years you'll know an awful lot about several dozen herbs.

ABOUT LATIN NAMES

Yeah, I know: They're a big pain in the brain. But if you're going to be serious about herbal medicine (and herbs in general), you'll just have to grit your teeth and learn Latin names. All medicinal uses are referenced to the Latin names of the plants so there won't be any (potentially) fatal mistakes. There are simply too many species and too many common names, and this can be confusing unless you are familiar with the Latin names.

For example, I know of at least a dozen plants that are called snakeroot in one place or another. In Kansas, echinacea (which is used to balance the immune system) is one of several plants known by that name. But I once had a traveling herbalist from Arizona try to sell me his local snakeroot, which was osha *(Ligusticum porteri)*, an herb used primarily for respiratory and intestinal problems. Had I purchased and used his snakeroot, my patients would have responded in an entirely different manner.

Insist on a Three-Book Minimum

If you are going to be serious about medicinal herbs, you'll need to own at least three good plant books. I own more than 500 herb books, and it seems I am constantly discovering some lovely little factoid about plants hidden within one of those books. And these little tidbits have ultimately helped me know — really know — the herbs.

Gone are the days when you couldn't find a decent herb book. Many of the herb books on the market today are good, if not excellent. (Of course, this is the best of the best, but that goes without saying!) However, no one book can be complete in all it says about herbs, and no book can contain a complete listing of all medicinal herbs. You will find invaluable information in almost any herb book, and some of that material you won't be able to find in any other book.

However, books often contradict one another. When two books don't agree, I know that I need to do more research to find out which of the two is right. For example, one book might say that an herb is perfectly safe, while another has three paragraphs of contraindications. In that case, I continue my research to weed out the incorrect information. I always wait until I have a thorough understanding of the herb before I use it on my patients.

Use It!

Now, there's book learning and there's real learning. Real learning is hands-on. Herbs are meant to be used. They were sent to Earth so we mortals could learn to heal our pets and ourselves by using the remedies we find in our own backyards.

Take it one herb at a time. Read about the herb and then apply your knowledge. See how your dog likes it. Mix up a tea and soak his food in it. Try sprinkling the chopped herb over his food. Offer a bit of tincture and see how he takes to it. And while your dog tries the herb, take it yourself and see how it affects you.

Get Your Hands Dirty

Most of the healing herbs mentioned in this book can be grown in your own backyard. There's no better way to be intimately connected to the healing powers of Mother Earth than when your hands are in the soil/soul of healing and you're getting dirty and sweaty while stretching, hoeing, pulling, and digging. Watch the herbs grow in the sun, and pick them for your family's use. You'll be learning all the while.

Let Nature Be Your Guide

Some of our most powerful healers are known to many as weeds. But weeds have much to teach us.

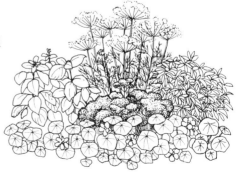

Tis Mal Crow, who is a Native American healer friend of mine, claims that he can tell which disease will enter a family and when by observing the plants growing around the family's household. "Yeah, right," I thought when I first heard the story.

But when I returned home to midtown Kansas City, I noticed a beautiful mullein plant growing in a neighbor's rock garden. It was the only mullein in the neighborhood, and I had tried, unsuccessfully, to grow the plant for years. So one afternoon I chatted with my neighbor about his new wife and mentioned how much I admired his wonderful mullein. He hadn't noticed the mullein; he thought it was just another weed. But he told me that his wife was in the hospital being treated for asthma — one of the primary diseases mullein is used to treat. Aha.

Watch the weeds in your backyard. Perhaps they are trying to teach you something.

LEARNING *FROM* THE HERBS

Mullein is a favorite herb of mine because, thanks to a herd of deer, it was the first plant to really teach me about medicinal herbs. One blustery, autumnal Kansas day, I watched as a small herd of deer feasted on a rangy weed in our backyard. After they had finished feeding, I took a weed identification book to the field and finally, after much searching, I identified the herb as mullein. I thought it strange for the deer to concentrate on one weed when there were still many other green plants around. Once I'd tasted mullein's fuzzy, stick-to-the-roof-of-your-mouth leaves, I wondered even more.

After a little more research into the medicinal properties of mullein, however, I understood that the deer were simply preparing their lungs for the cold wet weather to follow, and mullein was their protective herb of choice.

Make Your Herbal Studies FUN

Herbs — and herbalists — are a hoot. The more fun your studies, the more you'll learn.

Much like the soil they grow in, herbs are something you can really dig into. There's simply nothing more fascinating than herbs, and you can let your studies take you in whatever direction piques your interest. While this book focuses on medicinal applications of herbs in dogs, there are virtually endless options to whet your special-interest appetite. Enjoy the adventure.

Delivery Systems

Some dogs naturally take to the herbs they need. For those individuals, using a tea or bulk herb on the food or in the water is the best dosing method. Other dogs are not herb lovers, and they may need some additional coaxing. Capsules or tablets work well for stubborn critters, *if* you can get the pills down. (Many of them are horse-pill size!) Tinctures (especially the glycerin-based, nonalcoholic ones) are accepted by most pets, and a small dose — generally several drops, two or three times a day — is all that is needed.

The key is to use *whatever* herbal delivery method (bulk herbs, teas, tablets, capsules, or tinctures) works most easily for you and for your dog. Following is more information to help in your selection.

DOSAGE AND POTENCY

How much of the herb do I give and for how long? Well, if I were to look at the herbs as a "Western medicine man," I would want to know what quantity of a specific chemical is needed to counterattack the disease-causing biochemical entity that has invaded Rover's body. Using Western medicine's paradigms I would be evaluating a drug's *potency* by identifying its biochemical constituents and how those constituents affect individual cells.

Then my therapeutic approach would be to build up a blood level of the single-entity drug to a point where it would be effective in most (but certainly not all) patients, and I would continue giving that drug for a set amount of time. Many practitioners simply ignore the potential for adverse side effects of the drug, putting them into the "reasonable costs for the benefits rendered" category.

As a holistic practitioner who uses herbs, I view the disease and the cure entirely differently. First of all, I must remember that I am not using a single-entity drug that requires a specific blood level to be effective. Herbs have both synergy and bidirectionality working for them. Thus, from the perspective of therapeutic activity, trying to determine an herb's potency is nearly impossible, and it doesn't make much sense to try to do so by biochemical analysis. The most effective use of herbs is to activate and rejuvenate an organ system (or multiple organ systems), so I look for herbs — along with supplements, medications, and other factors — to help bring the animal's whole body back into balance.

How much herb it will take to activate that organ system depends on the herb and the animal. Each individual disease and animal will need a different amount of herbal content to return to normal health, or homeostasis.

Licorice

Dose to Effect

In light of all this, the easiest way to look at herbal dosages is to "give them to effect." My basic rule is to **start out slowly,** with low doses at first. Then, after a month or so, when the dog adjusts to her herbal intake, **taper off** or **add on,** depending on the dog's reaction.

Now, there are exceptions to this general rule, but in my practice they are few and far between. When treating a bacterial infection, for example, I might want to ensure that the blood level of active antibacterial ingredients is high enough to be effective. In this case I would be concerned about the "standardized" level of the antibacterials in the herb. But even with a bacterial infection, for the long term I am much more concerned about enhancing the immune system than I am about confronting the bacteria by outside means. (Interestingly, plenty of evidence indicates that while common Western antibiotics confront bacteria, they actually have an adverse effect on the patient's overall immune system.)

Building on these ideas, I offer here some other suggestions and strategies for combining herbs in different ways, depending on what is most acceptable to your dog:

- **Expect slow and easy results.** Herbs most often need to be given for at least 30 days before you'll see appreciable results. Look for mild and subtle — and long-lasting — changes.
- **Use the delivery system that works best (and most easily) for your dog.** It is more important to get the herbs into the dog's system than it is to worry about the "proper" way to dose.
- **Start out slowly and then, depending on the dog's reaction, taper off or add on.** Often, very small amounts of herb are enough to activate organ systems, ultimately leading to the cure you want.

GENERAL RULES FOR ADMINISTERING HERBS TO DOGS

Follow these guidelines to determine how much of an herbal preparation you should give your dog.

DOG WEIGHT	SPRINKLES (put on Pet's food once daily)	TEAS (pour over food or into Pet's water)	CAPSULES/ TABLETS	TINCTURES* (add to Pet's water or food or give directly by mouth)
1–10 lbs.	a small pinch	less than ¼ cup 1 to 3 times daily	½ capsule**, 1 to 3 times daily	1 to 3 drops, 2 or 3 times daily
10–20 lbs.	a bigger pinch	about ¼ cup, 1 to 3 times daily	½ to 1 capsule**, 1 to 3 times daily	3 to 5 drops, 2 or 3 times daily
20–50 lbs.	2 pinches to 1 teaspoon	¼ to ½ cup, 1 to 3 times daily	1 or 2 capsules**, 2 or 3 times daily	5 to 10 drops, 2 or 3 times daily
50–100 lbs.	2 pinches to 2 teaspoons	½ to 1 cup, 1 to 3 times daily	1 or 2 capsules**, 3 or 4 times daily	10 to 20 drops, 2 or 3 times daily
Over 100 lbs.	up to 1 tablespoon	up to 1 cup, 3 times daily	adult human dose	adult human dose

*1 dropperful = 20 to 30 drops
** or tablets

SELECTING HERBS

In my experience, the best benefits are obtained with top-quality whole herbs. Most important to me is that the herbs are organically grown; pesticides and herbicides can interfere with the healing properties of plants. I don't think there is a huge difference between fresh and dried herbs, especially when top-quality products are used.

A good herbal wholesale outlet has numerous levels of quality control to ensure that the plants sold are of the highest potency. A quality-control manager will conduct a physical examination of the herbs — look at them, smell them, feel them. He may also perform a chemical analysis, determine the spore content under a microscope, and even send a sample out for spectral chromatography. But it's just as important that the manager perform a simple taste test to ensure positive identification of the herb!

The best advice I can give for buying herbs is to find a source you trust and stick with it. There is a huge herb store not far from where I live, but I found out recently that the herbs are warehoused in a building that is regularly fumigated! On the other hand, I found an herbal outlet in Iowa (Frontier Herbs; see Resources) that offers plant materials that are consistently very fresh and well prepared. I now use that outlet for almost all my herbs, and when I know that a commercial product uses herbs from Frontier Herbs, I am comfortable that it contains quality plants.

What to Look For in Dried Herbs

When selecting dried herbs, I look for plants that are dry yet still resilient. If the plant is so brittle that it falls apart when you touch it, it's probably too old to be useful. I also look for plants that have retained a lot of color; properly dried green plants are still bright green. If the plants are brown and the leaves are crunchy, they are too old.

What to Look For in Fresh Herbs

When buying fresh herbs, select fresh-smelling plants that look healthy and have strong, green leaves. Avoid plants that are dusty, are browned, or have leaves with a moth-eaten appearance.

In addition, I often gather wild herbs for use on my animals and on me. You can do this too, but you *must* adhere to the following cautions:

- **Accurate identification is critical,** for obvious reasons. Most of the herbs I recommend are very common and easy to identify. But until you are intimately familiar with an herb, you should have an expert confirm your identification.
- **Be careful about harvesting herbs in urban and suburban environments,** which have most likely been treated with pesticides and herbicides. Even plants within a certain distance — some say 300 feet — from rural roads are not safe. Roadside plants, as well as herbs that grow near railroads and under high-voltage power lines, are typically sprayed with potent chemicals. Do not use an herb unless you are absolutely certain that it has not been sprayed.

How to Store Herbs

If you've purchased fresh herbs, use them within a few days; they will spoil eventually, just like food. If you've purchased dried herbs, you can store them for later use. Put your dried herbs in separate clean, glass jars and cap them tightly. Don't forget to label each jar with the name of the herb and the date you purchased it. If you keep the containers out of direct light and heat, the herbs will last for several months.

BULK HERBS

There are three ways to use bulk herbs:

1. Make a tea by simmering or steeping the fresh or freshly dried herbs in water.
2. Use tea bags as a more convenient way to make teas.
3. Sprinkle the bulk herb over your pet's food, much as you would add salt to your own.

When adding an herbal taste to Spot's food or water, be sure that she continues to eat and drink. In general, teas seem to be more readily accepted than sprinkles, at least at first.

Using Sprinkles

Many, but not all, dogs enjoy the taste of herbs. (I've discovered that cayenne, or red pepper, is a favorite seasoning for many of my patients, canine and feline.) Sprinkles can be made of fresh or dried herbs, and are best cut or ground into small pieces. Try the sprinkles on a small portion of your dog's food and see whether he selects or avoids that portion of the serving. Evidence suggests that it is important for the animal to taste the herb, evidently triggering other body systems

Use your dog's food to deliver herbal medicine in tea or sprinkle form.

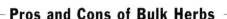

Pros and Cons of Bulk Herbs

There are big advantages to bulk herbs *if* your pet is accustomed to their taste:

- Low cost
- Ease of administration
- The "oral activating factor" (see above)
- The whole herb is present, adding the bidirectionality and synergistic effects (see page 20).
- There is no concentration of one ingredient with possible harmful doses present

There are also certain disadvantages:

- Not all health food stores carry bulk herbs
- Those that do may not pay attention to shelf life
- Some bulk herbs may have been sprayed (at the farm, warehouse, or distribution center) with potentially toxic pesticides
- Not all pets enjoy the taste, though I've learned that most adapt to the taste, given a few months

to actively accept the herb's healing properties. This is called the "oral activating factor."

Using Teas

After brewing tea with fresh or dried herbs (see recipe below for instructions) and then cooling the liquid, pour a small quantity onto your dog's food or into his or her water several times a day.

Don't let the herbalist jargon of tisane, decoction, and infusion befuddle you. If you're making a tea from thick, fibrous stuff, such as a root stalk, boil it a little harder and longer to make a **decoction.** If you're making your tea from fragile, sweet-smelling flowers or leaves, hold in that fragrance by covering your pot and boiling lightly. Voilà, you've made a **tisane** or **infusion.**

If you're a simple person from Kansas, like I am, you just boil some water, pour it over the plant stuff, and let it sit in a covered teapot until it has steeped for however much time you have available. Then, after you've had your cup of it and it has cooled down a mite, you give some to your pet.

Basic Herbal Tea

8 tablespoons fresh herb *or* 4 teaspoons freshly
   dried bulk herb *or* 2 herbal tea bags
1 quart boiling water

1. Simmer or steep the fresh or freshly dried bulk herb or tea bags for 10 to 20 minutes. Strain out the herb material and allow the liquid to cool.
2. Pour ¼ cup or so of tea over your dog's food two or three times a day, or add small amounts to his water.
3. Store the excess tea in the refrigerator to use over the next few days.

TINCTURES (A.K.A. LIQUID OR FLUID EXTRACTS)

These preparations are made by soaking the fresh or freshly dried herb in a solvent. In general, tinctures are considered more clinically effective than capsules or tablets.

There are two major solvents: alcohol and glycerin (or glycerite). For most herbs alcohol is the best solvent, extracting more of the plants' active ingredients than the other types of solvents. Alcohol, however, can be toxic in some patients, causing gastrointestinal irritation, allergic reactions, and (at least in people) habituation.

Nonalcoholic tinctures (which are often found on the shelves as "pediatric") are typically extracted in glycerin, a sweet-tasting solvent that can mask the taste of bitter herbs. Glycerin, which is available in most health food stores, is not quite as efficient as alcohol at extracting plant constituents, but it is a good alternative. Since the goal is to get a therapeutic amount of the herb into your dog, it might be more effective to feed her a larger amount of the weaker tincture.

If you have used fresh plants, you may find a gooey kind of scum — a viscous layer where the water and the oil haven't mixed — on the top of your extract. Don't worry a bit about it; there is nothing harmful about this layer. In fact, I know one herbalist who swears this gooey stuff is the most potent part of the tincture!

All you need to make a tincture is a clean jar with a tight-fitting lid, as much herb as it will take to fill the jar (fresh and dried herbs can be used with equal success), and either alcohol or glycerin to cover the herbs. For a tincture that will be stored and used for a couple of years, choose a substance that is at least 40 percent alcohol. Gin works fine, as does brandy. Some people use Everclear, a powerful alcohol, but the stronger the alcohol, the worse it will taste. A mild 20 percent alcohol may be used, but the resulting tincture won't last as long. That is fine, however, when the administration of the herb is expected to be short term.

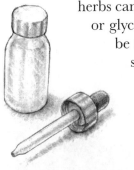
Tinctures are simple to make and keep for long periods of time.

Administering Tinctures

Tinctures can be used on your dog's food or in small amounts in his water. Or for the fastidious eater, you can use an eyedropper to squirt a few drops into his mouth or into the fold at the crease of his lips. Whenever possible, use the nonalcoholic tinctures. I have found that very small amounts — a few drops between the lower lip and gums at the side of the mouth two or three times daily, plus a few more drops in his water dish or atop the food — are often more than enough to be effective. Pet and praise and feed him a little treat afterward so that he will associate positive experiences with the administration of the tincture.

Simple Tincture

Fresh or dried herb of choice
Solvent of choice

1. Stuff a clean glass jar with the herb; leave an inch or two of space at the top. Fill the jar the rest of the way with the solvent.
2. Close the jar tightly and put it in a dark cupboard for a week or two. If the liquid is not very discolored with essences from the herb, let it soak a week or so longer. Shake the jar every few days.
3. Strain the plant material out of the liquid. Muslin or cheesecloth works best to capture all the little plant particles, and you can also use the cloth to squeeze as much liquid as possible from the plants. Rebottle the liquid and discard the plant material. Label the bottle with the date and the plant and solvent used. Alcohol tinctures can be kept for a long time (depending on the strength of the alcohol) in a cupboard; glycerin tinctures will keep longer in the refrigerator. Do not expose the tincture to direct heat or light.

GIVING A DOG A TINCTURE

Hold your dog securely. At the side of the mouth, gently pull down the lower lip.

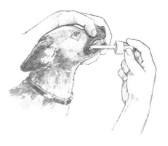

Use the eyedropper to squeeze a few drops of the tincture between the dog's lower lip and gum. The easiest place to do this is usually at the corner of the mouth right where the upper lip meets the lower lip.

Using Alcohol

There are only very small amounts of alcohol in a normal dose of an alcohol-tinctured herb for dogs, so I consider them generally safe for most patients. The actual amount of alcohol when several drops of herbal tincture are placed in as little as 4 ounces of water is less than 0.1 percent. A 12-ounce glass of beer contains, on average, 0.4 to 0.6 of an ounce of alcohol, while 6 dropperfuls of an average liquid herbal extract contain only 0.09 of an ounce.

The alcohol content can be reduced by simmering the extract in a small amount of water for 5 to 10 minutes. As a general rule, though, when you can find the prescribed herb in a nonalcoholic (glycerin) tincture, that is the preferred way to dose it. I recommend tinctures for the short term (a few weeks to months) when a patient has a specific problem that I feel can be helped by therapeutic levels of the herb.

CAPSULES AND TABLETS

There are two basic ways to make capsules and tablets:

1. Pack the powdered form of the herb (along with various fillers) into a capsule.
2. Use a tincture of the herb and soak it in the stuff that will make up the pill — powdered fillers and binders. Let the fluid portion of the tincture evaporate. What remains is a pill-tablet with the non-fluid portion of the tincture dissolved into the powdered components.

Capsules and tablets are inexpensive, and for the easy-to-pill pooch, they are convenient to give. On the downside: Adulteration may be a problem since the powdered forms are difficult to identify. Some capsules contain as much as 65 percent filler, such as soy or millet powder. And some commonly used binding agents include magnesium stearate, which can come from either animal or vegetable sources, and dicalcium phosphate, which may contain lead. It pays to know your herbal manufacturer and distributor.

Using Capsules and Tablets

If it is a product made for animals, read the label; if it is a made-for-human product, read the label and adapt the dosage to your dog's size (see the chart on page 35). Capsules and tablets are not my favorite way to administer herbs, but if they are the only way to get Pooch to take the medicine, then have at it. Rule #1 applies here: Whatever works.

TOPICAL HERBAL APPLICATIONS

There must be hundreds of topical herbal medicines on the market — oils, ointments, salves, soaps, and so forth. Skin is an animal's largest body organ, and it readily and actively absorbs all sorts of healing agents. Topical use of herbs, then, can be a highly effective delivery system for herbal healing.

We need to be a bit careful when using the topicals, however, because some of the carrying agents may be irritating to Pet's skin. Also, dogs will almost certainly lick off anything that is applied to their skin, and some of the carrying agents may cause intestinal upset.

How to Choose Topicals

"Natural-based" oils and salves — such as beeswax, lanolin, and coconut, olive, almond, grapeseed, and jojoba oils — are best and cause the fewest reactions. Petroleum-based and coal tar–based products seem to cause more reactions, and if the product label contains something you can't pronounce, don't use it. If your dog is especially sensitive to anything, use a test

GIVING A DOG A PILL

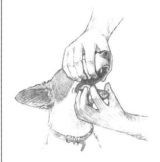

Straddle your dog and pull up on the top of the mouth with one hand.

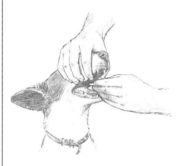

Place the pill on the very back of the tongue with your other hand.

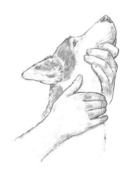

Hold the mouth shut with one hand while stroking the throat to encourage swallowing.

dose — a small amount applied to one area of your dog's skin — and watch her for 4 to 6 hours for signs of adverse reactions.

Making Your Own Topicals

My favorite topical application for wounds or other small areas is an herbal spritz. To give your dog a spritz, make the appropriate herb into a tea (see page 39 for instructions), allow it to cool, and spray it onto the area directly. Use this treatment three to five times a day. The spritzed herb will dry quickly, giving your dog little reason to lick. And even if the dog does lick, he or she ingests only the healing herb.

One longtime patient, a 13-year-old springer spaniel, began to lose his appetite. I found that the best way to treat this particular dog was to apply a few drops of an echinacea and goldenseal tincture directly to the fold of skin inside his lower lip.

Remember that because the herbs are absorbed so readily through the skin, a daily romp and roll in your herbal garden is one of the best ways to apply the healing qualities of herbs.

A special cautionary note: Individual herbal constituents of the essential oils used in aromatherapy may be concentrated to levels dozens of times higher than those found in the original herbs. With the altered levels of individual constituents, we may increase the possibility of adverse reaction, especially if your dog can lick and ingest the essential oil. So I limit topical application of essential oils to those herbs I know are nontoxic, and I apply only small amounts (a drop or two will do) to the rear of the dog's neck, just behind the ears.

USING AN HERBAL SPRITZ

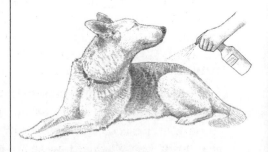

Spray the cooled infusion directly on the affected area.

STANDARDIZED EXTRACTS

Standardized extracts have been certified by the manufacturer — usually using a stringent laboratory method, such as liquid chromatography — to contain the stated amount of specific constituents. Standardizing may provide more consistency in potency and help ensure that the correct plant is being sold.

There are two types of standardized extracts:

- **Whole plant standardized extracts,** in which the entire plant is extracted and the plant's constituents are guaranteed to be above a certain level. For instance, a capsule might be guaranteed to contain exactly 1 milligram of the herb. But if only the amount of the herb present is guaranteed, you have no idea of the potency.
- **Purified standardized extracts,** which are herbal extracts made with a variety of solvents, with the active ingredient(s) removed from the parent plant. In this way, the original balance of the herb is significantly altered, as one constituent is "pumped up" above its normal levels. A St.-John's-wort capsule, for example, might contain 0.5 milligram of hypericin, which was once believed to be the herb's active ingredient. But this method assumes that the hypericin is the biochemical constituent that is needed, and the body may or may not get the benefits of the plant's other active ingredients, depending on whether they were extracted along with the hypericin.

There are plenty of out-to-make-a-buck-at-any-cost herbal hooligans, perfectly willing to extract your dollars for an inferior product. It is not uncommon to find herbal products on the market that do not contain (or that contain only minuscule amounts of) the herbs advertised on the package label. So some form of quality assurance is needed.

Are Standardized Extracts the Best Choice?

I am not so certain standardization is the answer. Any standardization process neglects the all-important healing factors involved in the synergistic actions of the *numerous* active ingredients of all herbal medicines. In addition, standardization typically looks at only the chemical properties of one part of the herb, again neglecting the possibility that the whole herb may have more potential value than is contained in its chemical constituents.

Finally, standardization does not take into account factors that may be important in the herb's potency and, thus, the overall healing properties — such as method of harvest, time of harvest, sex of the plant (or other individual conditions of the plant that indigenous healers thought were important), organic or commercial growing conditions, and so forth.

To my way of thinking, standardization is the lazy way of letting outsiders (the government) do what really should be the herbalist's groundwork of finding trustworthy herbal farmers, producers, suppliers, and distributors. Remember that when you grow (or gather in the wild) and make your own herbal medicines, *you* become the most trustworthy one. And you'll know that by using the whole herb, you won't alter the ratio of biochemicals naturally present and won't risk losing the synergy and bidirectionality of the plant.

ADAPTING HUMAN PRODUCTS FOR USE ON DOGS

If what you've purchased is a product meant for humans, read the label and adapt the directions to your dog's size. Assume that an average human weighs 150 pounds. Here are some examples of how this works.

Tinctures. The label instructions on the human product are to give 20 to 30 drops, three or four times a day, for a total daily human dose of 60 to 120 drops. Your dog weighs 15 pounds. 15 = 1/10 of 150 pounds, so the dog should receive 6 to 12 drops daily, preferably divided into three or four doses. A three-times-daily dosage, then, would be 2 to 4 drops.

Capsules or tablets. The label instructions for humans are to give 3 to 5 capsules, three times a day. If your dog weighs 30 pounds (30 lbs. = 1/5 of the "normal" 150-pound human), you could give up to 1 capsule or tablet three times a day. But if your dog weighs only 15 pounds, you could break the tablet in two (or open the capsule and use about half of its contents) and use this half capsule/tablet dosage three times daily.

Teas. Simmer fresh or dried bulk herb or an herbal tea bag (see recipe on page 39). The tea will last for a few days in the refrigerator. Add about 1/4 cup to your dog's food two or three times a day.

part 2

Herbs for Organs, Systems, and Special Conditions

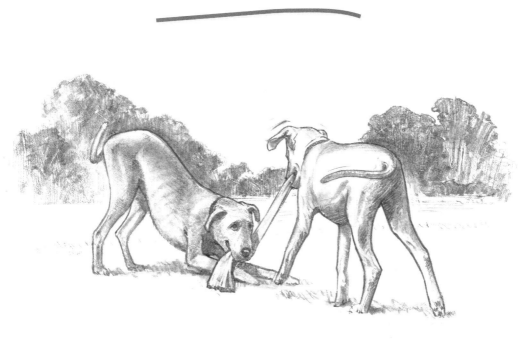

The Aging Body

As a 50-something graybeard, I have a lot of empathy for my aging dog, Rufus. He is almost as gray around the muzzle as I am, and I know exactly how his rusty joints feel when he gets up off his bed in the morning. Neither he nor I is quick to hear my wife, Sue, when she calls, and both of us are a little stockier around the middle — despite taking in almost exactly the same amount of daily food we ate when we were younger. He and I are both slower in our get-along, and neither of us sees as well as we once did. I understand perfectly that he just wants to lie by my side and be petted as I type away on this book.

The fact is that nearly all of Rufus's and my body systems are not what they once were. We cannot deny these age-related changes, but both of us are learning that herbal tonics are the perfect companions as we continue our journey through life.

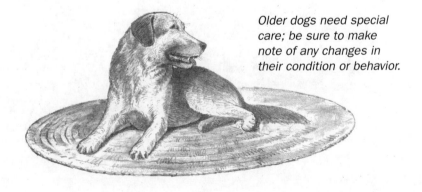

Older dogs need special care; be sure to make note of any changes in their condition or behavior.

A HOLISTIC PROTOCOL FOR AGING

Nothing can prevent aging, but you can prevent some of the problems associated with it. Rufus and I take our daily dose of herbs for one organ system or the other. We use several of my favorite herbs (many of which are listed in this book), concentrating on one organ system for a month or so and then moving on to another organ system. Both of us over the years have come to enjoy the tart taste of the herbs; indeed, neither of us enjoys our food quite as much without the tang of herbs sprinkled on top.

Use Tonic Herbs

Tonic herbs support the function of different organs, which, in turn, improves the overall health of the body. I prefer to use tonic herbs on an on-off basis, alternating them as our taste buds, our perceived needs for the month, and the availability of the herbs dictate. My favorite tonic herbs for the aging dog include:

- **Dandelion,** which enhances liver function and is a diuretic
- **Echinacea,** a general immune-system balancer
- **Ginger,** which boosts a lethargic digestive system
- **Hawthorn,** a cardiotonic that helps the aging heart
- **Milk thistle,** a liver-function enhancer
- **Nettle,** a gentle, whole-body tonic
- **Sarsaparilla,** a male rejuvenator and immune-system enhancer
- **Saw palmetto,** a male rejuvenator that is especially good to help avoid prostatic hyperplasia (enlargement)

Evaluating Aging Organ Systems

I recommend a special annual exam for healthy geriatric dogs, starting soon after they have passed their seventh or eighth birthday. Along with a regular physical exam, I suggest a complete blood count (CBC), a urinalysis, a series of blood chemistries, and possibly X rays. These exams are a way for me to screen for organ-related problems; catching these problems early, at a time when we can actually do something about them, is very important. The annual exam is the perfect way to identify organ systems that can be helped with herbs.

Get Adequate Exercise

I am a firm believer in the adage "Use it or lose it." So even though exercise is more of a chore than a pleasure for both Rufus and me, we make it a point to take our country walks at least four times a week. And while I lift weights to maintain the muscle mass that wants to deteriorate with every passing year, Rufus chases his ball for a daily muscle-building routine.

Incorporate Antioxidants

As we age, our cells are producing more and more free radicals — chemicals that speed the aging process. One of the keys to antiaging is to counter this overproduction of free radicals with antioxidants. Vitamins C and A are good antioxidants, but so are many herbs. Some of the culinary herbs even have antioxidant activity. These include:

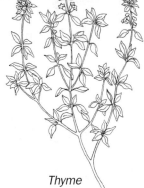

- Basil *(Ocimum basilicum)*
- Oregano *(Origanum vulgare)*
- Thyme *(Thymus vulgaris)*

Thyme

LONGEVITY HERBS?

In addition to the above regimen, both Rufus and I are gradually adding to our daily intake herbs that can enhance the length and quality of life during the golden years.

Ginkgo (Ginkgo biloba)

Ginkgo is our primary antiaging herb. It acts on two major systems of the body: the nervous system and the cardiovascular system. Ginkgo has proved effective in treating Alzheimer's disease, depression, and senile dementia. (In animals, senile dementia associated with Alzheimer's-like symptoms is referred to as cognitive dysfunction or dimming mind syndrome.) Ginkgo enhances both long-term and short-term memory in puppies and old critters alike. This popular herb improves circulation and has good antioxidant activity. Studies also indicate that ginkgo is often effective as treatment for age-related hearing and vision loss, dizziness and vertigo, and tinnitus (ringing in the ear).

Rosemary (Rosmarinus officinalis)

Rosemary contains bioactive ingredients that help prevent the breakdown of the chemical acetylcholine in the brain. A deficiency in acetylcholine is believed to be a contributing factor in senility in general and Alzheimer's disease in particular. Rosemary is also an important antioxidant.

> **R**ufus, my wife, and I all take our antiaging herbs on a daily basis, and I am firmly convinced that they are helpful. And judging by the comments from my many clients who are using the herbs I've recommended for their older dogs, herbs are truly one of the very best treatments available for the aging body.

Flaxseed Oil (Linum usitatissimum)

Flaxseed oil is an excellent source of omega-3 fatty acids, the good fats that reduce triglycerides and cholesterol (the prime fatty arterial blockers) and prevent blood clots.

Turmeric (Curcuma longa)

Turmeric is the yellow component of curry powder, and it stimulates the liver's bile production. This herb is a potent antioxidant. Turmeric is also heart healthy, acting as a blood thinner (which prevents clots) and helping to prevent excess cholesterol accumulation.

Green Tea (Camellia sinensis)

The green variety of tea contains flavonoids and polyphenols, which are a type of flavonoid that may be a more powerful antioxidant than vitamins C and E. Green tea is oxidized for a shorter period of time than black tea; practitioners don't think the black variety has the same health benefits.

Gotu Kola (Centella asiatica)

A traditional herb of both Chinese and Ayurvedic medicine, gotu kola has antioxidant activity that protects the body from damage by free radicals. The herb is particularly useful for stress-related disorders and memory problems. Rufus and I (and the rest of our aging family) are just beginning to try gota kola, so you should consult a local holistic practitioner to see if it will benefit your dog.

Arthritis and the Musculoskeletal System

Arthritis, and its cousin, rheumatism, encompass several dozen disease states of the joints and the surrounding tissues, such as tendons, ligaments, cartilage, joint sacs (or bursae), muscles, and connective tissues. Many conditions cause arthritis and rheumatism, including infection (bacterial, viral, fungal, and parasitic), trauma, immune-mediated diseases, old-age changes, orthopedic surgery, and genetic factors. Each of these causes has its own preferred method of treatment, so it is important to get an accurate diagnosis from your veterinarian.

THE MUSCULOSKELETAL SYSTEM

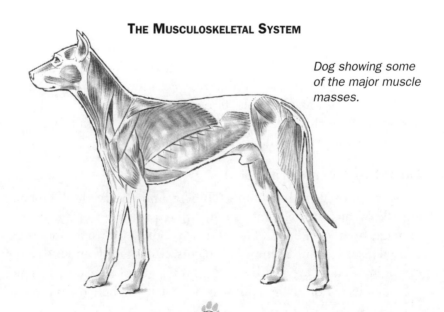

Dog showing some of the major muscle masses.

A Brief Introduction to Arthritis and Holistic Care

In my holistic practice in Kansas City, I treat more cases of arthritis than any other single disease. I have found that a holistic approach to the broad category of "arthropathies" is quite simply the best way to treat this multifaceted disease. I get much better results now than I ever did with Western medicines. I use a combined protocol of good nutrition, nutritional supplements, massage, passive exercise, acupuncture, chiropractic, and (of course!) herbs. Best of all, by applying a holistic approach, I see *far fewer* adverse side effects.

However, the same caveats apply foursquare when you use alternative medicines to treat arthritis or any other disease:

- Each and every case presents a different set of symptoms, and the individual patient's symptoms dictate which medicines should be used to try to effect a cure. In other words, there is no magic formula, herbal or otherwise, to treat all cases of arthritis.
- Alternative holistic methods do not typically work as fast as the whistle-and-bell Western medicines. Figure at least 2 months, and perhaps several different treatments, before you'll see any appreciable results; there is no quick fix in the alternative medicines. Remember that although it may take more time, in the long run your dog will have far fewer negative side effects.
- Each dog has a unique way of responding to treatments. And, unfortunately, I have never been able to predict from the onset which patients will be the ones to respond. Again, alternative medicines do not offer a quick fix or a magical formula.

Symptoms of Arthritis

The most common arthritic problems I see are a potpourri of osteoarthritic and degenerative arthropathies. Osteoarthritis is a joint disease that is characterized by degeneration of the articular cartilage, bone growth (bone spurs) at the edges of the joints, and changes in the synovial membrane that surrounds the joints.

Degenerative arthropathies are conditions characterized by deterioration of the joint cartilage, often accompanied by bone growth at the edges of the joints. Joint deterioration can be caused by trauma, infection, immune-mediated diseases, or developmental abnormalities. The typical patient is in mid- to old age (5 or more years old). The lower back and hips are the most commonly affected areas, but I've seen arthritis in every joint.

Most of the dogs I see have some form of genetic structural abnormality. Because of the way they are "put together," they constantly exert abnormal pressure on their joint surfaces, causing excess wear and tear and an increase of cell-produced free radicals. Wear and tear result in erosion of the joint's cartilage. Without the cushioning cartilage, bones may rub together, causing the dog pain. As the cartilage erosion progresses, bony growths may form, causing even more pain when your dog moves the joint.

Free radicals are atoms or groups of atoms that can cause damage and eventually death to cells. Small amounts of free radicals are formed by the normal metabolism of cells, and these are scavenged naturally in the body. However, when excess free radicals are formed, exceeding the body's ability to scavenge them, they attach to cell membranes and eventually cause cellular death. In their attack on cells, free radicals have been implicated in the following health problems: arthritis, premature aging, cancer, chronic degenerative diseases, immune-mediated diseases, heart disease and atherosclerosis (in humans), birth defects, and genetic mutations.

Typically, the symptoms slowly get worse until the dog has a difficult time getting up stairs or jumping onto Mom's bed. Perhaps your dog prefers to lie around in the warm sun and groans when getting up or lying down. There may be enough pain and inflammation in the joints that you see a noticeable limp when the dog walks; sometimes the joints are actually swollen. X rays may or may not show noticeable changes in the joints or bony surfaces, but a chiropractic evaluation will reveal joints that are less flexible than normal.

From the get-go I tell folks to figure a minimum of 3 months of treatment before we'll see any appreciable results. But once we do see results, they can be long lasting, and we will not use any drugs that are actually damaging to the dog's body.

Step One: Acupuncture and Chiropractic

I feel that acupuncture and chiropractic are essential elements in any treatment regimen for arthritis. Typically, after several initial treatments the dog exhibits much less pain, and we almost always see partial or nearly complete return of function. I see such good results from acupuncture and chiropractic that I think it is just plain bad medicine, perhaps even malpractice, not to use them.

Step Two: Nutrition

Often a change in diet is enough to relieve arthritic symptoms. Feed your dog good-quality, organic foods that are not overprocessed and contain no synthetic preservatives, pesticides, herbicides, hormones, or artificial flavors or colorings. Home-cooked is best.

Parsley

Step Three: Supplements

There is a veritable stewpot of supplements that have worked seemingly miraculous results in some patients with arthritis. The two most important categories of these are the antioxidants and chondroprotective agents.

Antioxidants protect cells from damage caused by free radicals. Free radicals are produced when a cell is exposed to any of a number of toxins, including pesticides, herbicides, and toxic emissions in the air. Free radicals are also produced by cells surrounding the joint whenever excess or abnormal strains and pressure are applied — for example, when the weight-bearing surfaces are out of normal alignment because of a skeletal disfigurement. To put antioxidants to work on the disease, I add therapeutic (i.e., high) levels of vitamins A, C, and E along with selenium to the dog's diet for 3 to 6 months, and then decrease the dosage to protective levels. Check with your holistic vet for the proper dosage, which should be adjusted for both the dog's size and the severity of the disease.

Herbal antioxidants. Many herbs are highly antioxidant and also contain good levels of necessary vitamins. I especially like the culinary herbs, such as oregano *(Origanum vulgare)*, thyme *(Thymus vulgaris)*, ginger, basil *(Ocimum basilicum)*, parsley *(Petroselinum crispum)*, and celery seed *(Apium graveolens)*, because they can be sprinkled on

OTHER ANTIOXIDANTS

In addition to the antioxidants listed on page 55, several others may prove helpful, including:

- Glutathione peroxidase
- Methionine
- Pycnogenol
- SOD (superoxide dismutase)

Other nutrients that have shown some promise in treating arthritis include:

- Boron
- Copper
- Magnesium
- Manganese
- Niacin (vitamin B_3)
- Pyridoxine (vitamin B_6)
- Zinc

The omega-3 fats — from deep-sea fish, flaxseed oil *(Linum usitatissimum),* and purslane *(Portulaca oleracea)* — may also be helpful.

your dog's food daily — much as you would season your own dinner. Find a combination of these herbs (along with cayenne and turmeric; see step 5 for more information) that your dog will eat. It's been my experience that unless the dog has become completely spoiled with the pap that characterizes typical commercial pet foods, he or she will enjoy one or more of these culinary treats.

Chondroprotective agents promote new cartilage growth and thus decrease pain and improve joint mobility. Glucosamine HCl products have generally given my patients the most consistent results. Other chondroprotective agents I have tried include chondroitin sulfate, MSM (methylsulphonylmethane), and SAM-e (S-adenosylmethionine). I add these to my protocol when glucosamine hasn't seemed to work after a few months' trial. I use the regular human dosage schedule, altered to fit my animal patient's weight (see chart on page 35).

Step Four: Exercise and Massage

I am of the "Use it or lose it" school of thinking, and the research on arthritis supports this approach. The more you can keep your dog moving and flexing her joints, the better. A daily walk on grass or some swimming (considered a passive exercise) can greatly retard the progress of arthritis. For many dogs with arthritis, however, even light exercise can be painful. See step 5 for some herbal treatments that may help.

A daily light massage can ease some of the aches and pains of this disease, as well as increasing general body circulation. See Resources for suggested books on this topic.

Step 5: Herbal Pain Relief

Both pain and inflammation are the common results of arthritic changes in the joint. But because it is most important to keep your dog "on the go" (see above), we need to do

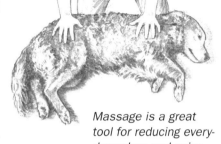

Massage is a great tool for reducing everyday aches and pains.

all we can to make your pet comfortable while moving. Herbs can be very helpful in relieving arthritis-related symptoms.

Licorice root *(Glycyrrhiza glabra)* is an herb I commonly use to replace the anti-inflammatory action of the steroids that I once used in my Western medicine practice. (We have a saying in Western veterinary medicine: "No animal should die without having been treated with cortisone." So Western vets [including me in my past life] use steroids for *everything*.) It's nice to have a nontoxic option to steroids, so many of my patients receive licorice root. It may take a month or two before your dog displays positive results, but he or she will avoid the adverse side effects of cortisone.

I am not convinced that we ever see in our animals the high-blood-pressure problems we see in people who take prolonged, high doses of licorice root. But to be honest, we never measure blood pressure in dogs, so I can't be sure. I can say that I have used the herb on hundreds of dogs and cats, many with preexisting heart problems, and I haven't seen any cardiac or renal problems.

Cayenne *(Capsicum* spp.), taken internally, seems to offer pain relief for some patients. In addition, cayenne acts as a systemic stimulant, helping move herbs and other medicines into joint areas where they are needed. I am surprised how many of my animal patients (both dogs and cats) enjoy the taste of cayenne sprinkled over their food, making this herb a great treatment option. For people, cayenne is also used topically as an ointment; it is applied directly over painful joints. However, our canine critters often go crazy trying to lick everything off their hair and skin, so they aren't usually good candidates for topical ointments that cause stinging.

Other valuable herbs are:

- Feverfew *(Tanacetum parthenium),* an excellent herb for the type of arthritis or rheumatism in which muscle pain is involved
- St.-John's-wort *(Hypericum perforatum),* which eases pain and speeds the healing process, especially of damaged nerves
- Wild yam *(Dioscorea villosa),* which is reported to be good for painful arthritis since it has actions similar to those of cortisone
- Willow bark *(Salix* spp.), which is rich in the anti-inflammatory salicylates, the stuff found in aspirin

Many of our "engineered" dog breeds are genetically predisposed to arthritic conditions. Look at a wolf, coyote, or fox. These critters have evolved without human intervention, so their skeletal structures are able to withstand the rigors of a normal day's activity. Now look at the bred-to-look-funny-or-cute dog breeds; you'll see how far from "normal" or "natural" they really are. The more structurally removed a dog is from a fox, coyote, or wolf, the nearer the animal is to the abnormal limbs and skeletal structure that predispose him or her to arthritic changes later in life.

Step 6: Herbs for Arthritis

Herbs are greatly helpful additions to the other alternative-medicine treatments. The key here is to match the herbal prescription to the critter and his or her particular form of arthritis. This is not always an easy task; references cite more than a hundred herbs that have been effective for someone's arthritis, and no one herb will work for all cases of the disease.

Some of my favorite herbs for arthritis include:

Alfalfa *(Medicago sativa)* and **yucca root** *(Yucca* spp.), herbs that have traditionally been used to treat arthritis. In fact, alfalfa may be one of the best of the traditional herbal treatments, with 10 percent of humans treated responding well and others gaining partial relief. The best part of these two herbs is that they can be grown in your own backyard.

Alfalfa

Devil's claw *(Harpagophytum procumbens)*, an herb from South Africa, which is a potent anti-inflammatory and a specific for treating arthritis and rheumatism.

Frankincense *(Boswellia* spp.), another herb traditionally used for arthritis. Like turmeric, frankincense is a popular arthritis treatment in Ayurvedic medicine.

Turmeric *(Curcuma longa)*, an anti-inflammatory herb that has been effectively used as a specific for arthritis in Ayurvedic medicine and other practices. Many dogs like the taste of turmeric.

I prefer to sprinkle arthritis herbs over the dog's dinner. This type of administration gives your dog the benefit of all of the herb's "inner medicines" and offers more safety than herbal extractions (tinctures), which may contain potentially toxic concentrations of one biochemical. However, some of the specific arthritic herbs — such as devil's claw, frankincense, and turmeric — may have an increased medicinal action when they are used in the concentrated doses found in tinctures, capsules, and tablets. In these cases, I use the human dose listed on the product label, adjusted to the dog's size.

Be Patient

Let me repeat my original word of caution: Do not expect significant results from an alternative treatment for 60 to 90 days. Assume that you may need to try several supplements and/or herbs until you find the proper mix for your pet. And resign yourself to the fact that your dog will most likely need those special supplements and herbs for the rest of his life. Remember that you've chosen the wisest and safest treatment possible.

Allopathic Drugs

In my opinion and in the opinions of other alternative-medicine practitioners who have studied the literature on allopathic medicines, the most common Western drugs used for inflammation and pain — steroids, salicylates (aspirin and aspirin substitutes), and nonsteroidal anti-inflammatory drugs (NSAIDs) — are definitely *contraindicated* for treating arthritis. Long-term use (for more than a couple of weeks) of any of these drugs causes nasty side effects, such as stomach ulcers and liver and kidney problems. In addition, the drugs actually inhibit the healing of joint surfaces, tendons, and ligaments. What's even worse, many of them also promote the degeneration of the joint-surface cartilage — the very process we are trying to prevent and heal.

Cancers

I love the media-generated image of one of my heroes, John Wayne, limping out to the front steps of the hospital where he'd just survived cancer therapy and growling in his wonderful, bulldog-raspy voice, "Well, boys, I've just whupped the Big C."

That's the spirit I want all my cancer clients to have: "Well, boys, I know my dog can whup the Big C. And he will do it with a John Wayne swagger of confidence." You see, I know full well that a positive mental attitude is a proven cancer antidote. I believe in miracles, and I think it helps when my clients do also. But because I'm a Midwestern country boy with an overload of pragmatism, I don't want any of my clients to think I have discovered *the* miracle cure for anything. And Lord knows, as I write this, I'm at least a chapter or two away from discovering the cure for cancer.

UNDERSTANDING CANCER

When I am presented with a dog that has cancer — any cancer — I have a few visuals that I think are helpful. I visualize the cancer cells as a group of rebellious teammates that have decided to play ball their own way, without regard for the rules of the game or the benefit of the other members of the team (the other cells of the body). These anti-team members, if allowed to grow in size and number, will eventually steal enough from the rest of the team (the rest of the body) to kill it. It's my job as a holistic veterinarian to rein in the rebellious cells and convince them that they should once again function as good team members.

Another way I look at cancer is as a lack of internal balance. A healthily functioning body works in balance: All organ systems perform their duties harmoniously and as needed. When healthy, the animal's body, mind, heart, and spirit are also in a natural state of balance. Cancer is the ultimate disease of imbalance. When cancer appears, something within the intricate homeostatic mechanisms of the dog's body has gone totally awry. If we are to "whup the Big C," we need to help your dog's body regain its state of natural homeostasis. When this happens, all the organ systems will be functioning properly, and the dog's body, mind, heart, and spirit will once again be balanced.

Where Do Herbs Fit In?

I don't expect herbs to perform anticancer miracles. I think the best way to use them in cancer patients is as organ-system balancers — improving the function of organs under attack by cancer cells and enhancing overall body mechanisms to give the dog's body its best chance to recover. Then, I always hold out that glimmer of hope that one of the herbs I select will be the one a particular patient needs, along with the other therapies I am recommending, to "whup the Big C."

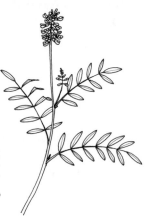

Astragalus

ANTICANCER PROTOCOL

My final piece of wisdom on cancer therapy is that the best long-term results I have seen have come when we go beyond thinking in terms of a single, magic cure and develop a complete program of holistic health. I use my 10-Step Protocol (see chapter 2) because it gives me a basis for a complete system of holistic care. In addition to that, my special anticancer protocol includes the following:

1. Develop a positive belief system.
2. Eliminate as many potential causes of cancer as possible.
3. Add nutritional and supplemental support.
4. Use classical homeopathy.
5. Incorporate herbs that enhance organ function (and possibly act as an anticancer therapy).

Step 1: Develop a Positive Belief System

Use your best John Wayne swagger to create and maintain a positive attitude. Prayer, whatever your religious affiliation, has been proved to help in the healing process. Don't underestimate the power of this step.

Step 2: Eliminate All Potential Causes of Cancer

Go through your dog's entire environment. Modify it so that he or she avoids contact with pesticides, herbicides, airborne pollutants, and toxic household chemicals found in the carpets, in the furniture, under the sink, and in the garage. Give your pet filtered water, and serve water and food in nonplastic (ceramic or glass) dishes.

Step 3: Add Nutritional and Supplemental Support

Perhaps the most effective component of any cancer cure is to put your dog on a good diet. Home-cooked organic foods are best. There are other health foods commercially available that do not contain preservatives, and they are made from mostly organic (or hormone-, antibiotic-, pesticide-, and herbicide-free) high-quality foods.

Supplements are an excellent addition to a quality diet. Use therapeutic levels of antioxidants — vitamins A and C and the culinary herbs — and add extra levels of zinc, selenium, and omega-3 fatty acids (flaxseed).

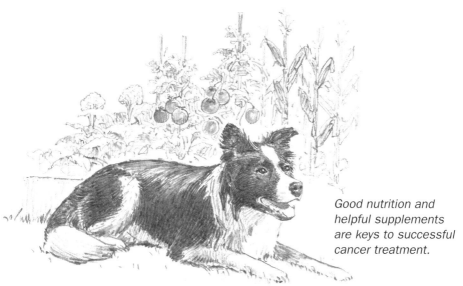

Good nutrition and helpful supplements are keys to successful cancer treatment.

Miracles

I believe in miracles, I really do. I have to; by using alternative medicines, I see miracles almost every day. But I tell all my clients: I do not know of any alternative treatment, herbal or otherwise, that will work for all cancers, every time. Whenever I think I have found an herb that is always (or even most of the time) effective, the very next patient proves me and my chosen herb wrong.

I cringe whenever I hear of someone who claims to have found a cancer cure. I call such people Cancer Charlatans. They are often well-meaning folks who have seen a cancer case (or several) respond favorably to some magical formula, but they have not tried their magic on enough patients to know that it will not work on everyone. Some are simply money grubbers with a financial interest in some foo-foo dust that they can sell to clients who are desperate for a cure.

I consider many of the proponents of Western medicine's approach to cancer therapy to be Cancer Charlatans, too. I think that when they talk to clients, they tend to overestimate the percentage of cancer cases that are cured long term by surgery, chemotherapy, or radiation therapy. But what's even worse, they often grossly underestimate the likelihood of severe adverse side effects from their methods.

I tell all my cancer clients to hope and pray for a miracle. I am also comfortable telling them that many, but not all, animals have a fair to good response to alternative therapies. Most of my patients even seem to enjoy a decent quality of life while they are undergoing therapy, a direct contrast to those undergoing chemo and radiation therapies. I advise my clients that alternative therapies are typically slow — often taking several months before they begin to produce a positive response. Finally, I am the first to admit that some cases have not responded to anything I've tried, and, unfortunately, I have never been able to predict which dogs will respond and which will not.

Step 4: Use Classical Homeopathy

I have not found any medicine as powerful as classical homeo-pathy . . . when it works. With classical homeopathy you need to find the one remedy that best connects with the patient's totality of symptoms, and finding this one remedy can be a challenge. (I occasionally use acupuncture for some cancers, but homeopathy is most often my alternative treatment of choice.) Consult a holistic vet for the proper treatments.

Step 5: Incorporate Herbs to Enhance Organ Function

When the organ systems are balanced, the body is better able to fight cancer. The major herbs I use are those that enhance organ-system function, aiding the organs that are under attack by the cancer cells. For more information on herbs for the different body systems, refer to chapters 6–21.

HELPFUL HERBS

Many herbs have been used successfully to treat various cancers, and I have tried most of them at one time or another. Sometimes they work, sometimes not — it seems to be an entirely individual matter. But because many of the plants also enhance organ-system function, they are well worth trying.

Aloe (Aloe vera)

The juice of the leaves has been used internally to stop the spread (metastases) of tumors, although it apparently does not affect the main tumor growth.

Aloe

Astragalus (Astragalus spp.)

In addition to enhancing the immune system, Astragalus contains an alkaloid (swainsonine) that inhibits the spread of melanoma, a skin cancer.

Chaparral (Larrea spp.)

This herb contains a bioactive ingredient (nordihydroguaiaretic acid, or NDGA) that has shown antitumor activity in the mammary glands of rats. NDGA has also been used as a commercial antioxidant in fats and oils, and chaparral contains flavones. Both the flavones and NDGA's antioxidant activity are possible agents for chaparral's anticancer mode of action.

Echinacea (Echinacea *spp.*)

This important herb doesn't treat the cancer itself, but it exerts an indirect cancer-prevention action by balancing the immune system. The health of the immune system is key to the health of the body.

Garlic (Allium sativum)

This common herb has many sulfur-containing compounds, which are helpful in enhancing the immune system. One of these compounds, diallyl sulfide, has been shown to inhibit chemically caused cancers of the stomach and lungs in mice. Research also indicates that garlic stimulates the growth of beneficial cells. The consumption of the plant is associated with reduced deaths from cancer. However, recent research indicates that garlic causes a particular type of anemia in animals, especially in cats, so I am very cautious with its use.

Siberian Ginseng (Eleutherococcus senticosus)

Not to be confused with *Panax ginseng,* Siberian ginseng has been linked to inhibited tumor growth in rats. It is also a potent enhancer of the immune system.

Green Tea (Camellia sinensis)

One of those herbs that seem to have unlimited potential, green tea is a stimulant and immune-system booster. It's also an antioxidant and an astringent, and it has been shown to combat some stomach and skin cancers.

Pau d'Arco (Tabebuia *spp.*)

A tea made from the inner bark of this South American tree has been reported to have antitumor activity in some animals.

The Best of the Rest

Many, many herbs have been used traditionally to treat cancers, and it is often difficult (or impossible) to separate the glowing claims from the facts. I look at it this way: If the herb has otherwise useful activities, why not use it in the hope that it will treat this particular cancer? If, on the other hand, the herb has many negative side effects, then I am much more cautious. My main safe-to-use herbs include:

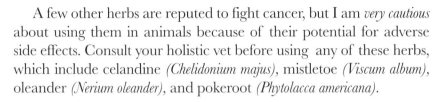

Red clover

- Bloodroot *(Sanguinaria canadensis)*
- Burdock *(Arctium lappa)*
- Cat's claw *(Uncaria tomentosa)*
- Goldenseal *(Hydrastatis canadensis)*
- Noni juice *(Morinda citrifolia)*
- Red clover *(Trifolium gratense)*

A few other herbs are reputed to fight cancer, but I am *very cautious* about using them in animals because of their potential for adverse side effects. Consult your holistic vet before using any of these herbs, which include celandine *(Chelidonium majus)*, mistletoe *(Viscum album)*, oleander *(Nerium oleander)*, and pokeroot *(Phytolacca americana)*.

Essiac

Essiac is an herbal cancer therapy developed by a Canadian nurse, Renée Caisse. *(Essiac* is *Caisse* spelled backward.) It is controversial; researchers have not been able to prove that it has any anti-tumor activities. However, thousands of people have claimed that it effectively treated their cancers, and some of my clients claim to have had great success with it in their dogs. Essiac contains burdock root, Chinese rhubarb *(Rheum palmatum)*, sorrel *(Rumex acetosa)*, and slippery elm *(Ulmus rubra)*.

Hoxsey Therapy

This combination of herbs has been in use as an unconventional cancer treatment for nearly 100 years. Harry Hoxsey, its developer, claims to have gotten parts of the formula from his grandfather and to have then learned the others from observing the plants one of his horses ate, apparently to cure itself of a life-threatening illness. Hoxsey Therapy uses a basic solution of cascara sagrada *(Rhamnus purshianus)* and potassium oxide plus one or more of the following herbs: pokeroot *(Phytolacca americana)*, burdock root, barberry *(Berberis* spp.), buckthorn bark *(Rhamnus frangula)*, stillingia root *(Stillingia sylvatica)*, and prickly ash bark *(Zanthoxylum americanum)*.

The Cardiovascular System

The cardiovascular system is an incredible, almost magical, mechanical wonder. Think about it. The system's workhorse is a pump that pulsates day and night throughout a dog's lifetime, beating consistently at the rate of 100 to 130 beats per minute (depending on the size of the dog; typically, the larger the animal, the slower the heart rate). This pump would fit in the palm of your hand, but it is capable of sending gallons of blood through a miles-long labyrinth of outbound arteries and returning veins.

But the heart and its supporting network of vessels are more than a *mechanical* wonder. In many cultures, the heart also holds a mysterious, almost mystical quality. In our culture, for example, we believe our heart when it tells us we have fallen in love. We "open our hearts" to those we trust. And we are "heartbroken" when someone close to us dies.

In Chinese medicine, the heart is seen as the center of consciousness, feelings, and thoughts. It houses the spirit of *Shen;* the Chinese written character for Shen can be translated as spirit, soul, God, godly, and effectiveness. The meaning of this principle is touched upon when one says that an animal has spirit. Dogs with mental imbalances of hysteria, such as an animal that panics and barks crazily, inexplicably paces, or bites out of fear, has a problem with heart Shen. Some seizure patterns are also attributable to heart imbalances.

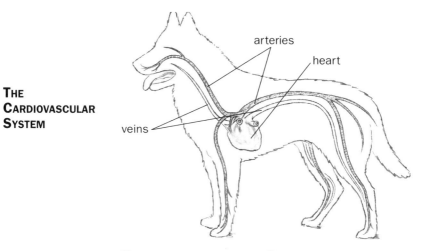

THE CARDIOVASCULAR SYSTEM

DISEASES OF THE CARDIOVASCULAR SYSTEM

The heart may be almost unbelievably powerful, but it can develop problems. Symptoms that may indicate heart disease in dogs include:

- Coughing
- Difficulty breathing
- Fainting
- General weakness
- Intolerance of exercise

When the veterinarian suspects heart disease, he or she places a stethoscope over the dog's chest and listens for any one of a multitude of irregular sounds. Heart murmurs, slowed or quickened heart rate, fibrillation, premature beats, lung congestion, and other symptoms may indicate that something is amiss within the system. Further tests might include electrocardiography, X rays, ultrasound evaluation, blood chemistry analysis, and heartworm tests.

What Are the Causes?

Cardiovascular disease may have infectious, mechanical, nutritional, hormonal, or parasitic causes. Here are some of the most common culprits:

- **Bacterial infections** often find residence in the heart's valves, causing initial mechanical obstruction with possible latent damage to the valves themselves.
- **Canine parvovirus** often infects the heart muscles, and the resulting death of muscle cells can sometimes result in acute heart failure.

- **Heartworms** can mechanically block the valves, and if enough are present they can clog an entire heart chamber.
- **Hormones,** especially of the thyroid, also affect heart function; hypothyroid dogs may have a slower than normal heart rate.
- **Nutritional deficiencies,** such as a lack of vitamin E or selenium, may damage heart muscles.

The primary causes of cardiovascular disease in humans, arterial cholesterol deposits and arteriosclerosis, are only very rare problems for our dogs. Specific therapy for any cardiovascular disease will, of course, depend on the diagnosis, but herbal medicines can be used to aid whatever therapy is used.

By far the most prevalent cause of heart disease in dogs is congenital — birth defects of the valves, vessels, and nerves that regulate the heart's ability to pulse naturally. Herbs offer the perfect mild, supportive care without appreciable adverse side effects. In fact, I've found the holistic/herbal approach to congenital abnormalities to be simpler and just as effective — if not more effective — than Western medicine's whistle-and-bell drugs.

A Holistic Treatment Plan

My holistic regimen for helping dogs with cardiovascular system diseases hinges on a four-pronged approach:

1. Herbs specific for the heart.
2. Diuretics. Because a diseased heart cannot pump blood properly, many patients with cardiac disease have concurrent congestion of the lungs. Diuretics help eliminate the excess fluids.
3. Other herbs that are supportive for the cardiovascular system.
4. Nutritional supplements.

SPECIFIC HERBS

Heart-specific herbs work in several ways, depending on the herb. They may:

- Have a normalizing effect on cardiac output — either depressing or stimulating its action (depending on the need)
- Dilate coronary vessels, thus improving the blood supply to the heart

- Have an overall anabolic effect on metabolism, creating a decrease in oxygen consumption and energy use
- Normalize cardiac rhythm
- Inhibit platelet aggregation (blood clotting)

Hawthorn (Crataegus laevigata)

This plant is quite simply the best heart medicine available. It acts as a cardiac tonic, normalizing the heart's activity by either depressing or stimulating its action (depending on the need). Therefore, hawthorn is good for heart failure or weakness, for heart palpitations, and as a general tonic for the circulatory system.

Hawthorn works by dilating vessels, including coronary arteries, and thus enhancing the metabolic processes in the heart muscles and improving blood supply to the heart and the rest of the body. It has an overall anabolic effect on metabolism; the herb creates a decrease in oxygen consumption and energy use. This means that when the heart is under stress, hawthorn helps improve its capacity for work. Hawthorn also abolishes some types of rhythmic disturbances. In addition, it has a mild diuretic effect and has been used traditionally as an anti-inflammatory herb.

For the great majority of cardiovascular problems I see in dogs, I recommend herbal medicines along with nutritional supplements and moderate exercise. In my opinion, these three therapies are the treatments of choice.

Like most herbs, hawthorn does not work quite as fast as some allopathic drugs, so it is not to be used for emergencies such as fibrillation. However, hawthorn has a synergistic effect with the drug digitalis; when the two are used in combination, the necessary digitalis dose may be about half of that normally prescribed. Compared with digitalis, hawthorn is safer and milder in activity — there is not a cumulative effect (an increased effect due to an accumulation of the drug in the body) with hawthorn, and hawthorn may actually decrease some of the adverse side effects of digitalis.

Almost no toxicities have been reported with hawthorn, but you should still check with a qualified herbalist before you combine hawthorn with other cardiac drugs.

Motherwort (Leonurus cardiaca)

This cardiac tonic is also used as a sedative and as a female-hormone normalizer. It is an excellent tonic for the heart, strengthening the muscle without making it strain. Motherwort is especially good for conditions in which the heart rate is increased because of anxiety and tension. The herb works by improving the metabolism of the heart muscles, reducing heart rate, increasing coronary perfusion (blood flow to the heart through the coronary arteries), and inhibiting platelet aggregation (clot formation).

For the female dog, motherwort is used to help prepare the uterus for pregnancy. During delivery, the herb can be used to promote contractions. Since motherwort promotes uterine contractions, it should not be used during the midphases of pregnancy.

Motherwort is generally free of toxicities, but some people may develop contact dermatitis from handling it.

Motherwort

DIURETIC HERBS

An animal with a heart that is not working up to snuff often has an accumulation of fluids throughout the body (referred to as edema, or ascites). These excess fluids can be especially evident in the lungs, where they can be heard with a stethoscope as fluid sounds (or rales). The lung-accumulated fluids often cause a persistent cough. Diuretic herbs make the animal urinate more frequently, helping eliminate these excess fluids.

Dandelion Root (Taraxacum officinale)

Dandelion is my favorite herbal diuretic. It is a potent one, but it is also liver supportive. Many Western medicine diuretics deplete potassium, which has an adverse effect on all muscles — especially heart muscles. Dandelion is a rich source of potassium, replacing the amount lost in the urine.

Other Diuretics

Other diuretics that you may want to consider include:

- Cleavers, which is also good for lymphatic swellings, dry skin conditions, and urinary tract infections
- Motherwort, which is specific for the heart, for calming anxiety, and for female reproductive problems
- Parsley, which is also a hypotensive and is good for liver and gallbladder problems
- Yarrow, which is used for fevers, infections, and liver and gallbladder problems

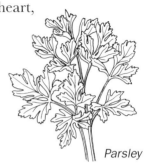

Parsley

Supportive Herbs

While the supportive herbs may not have a specific action on the heart, they are important for other reasons. For example, cayenne is a general tonic and has systemic stimulative effects. In addition, it helps regulate blood flow, making it a good herb to use to deliver other herbs to the areas of the body where they can do the most good. Supportive herbs all have beneficial effects for the different body systems.

Cayenne (Capsicum *spp.*)

This herb can be extremely helpful for the cardiac patient because of its systemic stimulant effect. It is a general tonic, specific for the circulatory and digestive systems. Cayenne regulates blood flow, equalizing and strengthening the heart, arteries, capillaries, and nerves. Since it is a general stimulant, I also consider cayenne good for helping deliver other herbs and nutrients throughout the body.

Ginger (Zingiber officinale)

Well known as an aid for digestive problems, ginger is also used as a stimulant for peripheral circulation. In addition, ginger acts as a diaphoretic, promoting perspiration.

Ginseng (Panax *spp.*)

Panax is another good example of an herb with bidirectional effects: Some of its compounds increase heart rate if needed; others decrease heart rate when indicated. Ginseng enhances physical vitality and can be especially helpful for an older dog that is weak or exhausted, or for a depressed dog.

NUTRITIONAL SUPPLEMENTS

If your dog has cardiovascular problems, he or she should be on a low-sodium diet. Include a moderate amount of daily exercise, without undue stress, strain, or overexertion. Nutritional supplements can also be helpful. Consider the following:

- Vitamins A, B_6, C, and E; folic acid; and the vitamin-like compound carnitine; these antioxidants help prevent damage from free radicals
- The minerals selenium and magnesium, which improve heart function
- Fatty acids, which can be supplied through flaxseed oil (omega-3 fatty acids) or evening primrose or borage oil (primarily omega-6 fatty acids), protect heart muscle cells

Whether or not to use one of the supplements listed above depends on each individual case. But the one supplement I almost always prescribe for heart problems is coenzyme Q_{10}, as it is almost specific for cardiovascular diseases. This potent antioxidant improves heart muscle oxygenation, and in people it seems to protect against heart attacks.

The Ears

Dogs frequently contract otitis externa, or external ear infection. This condition is caused by a wide variety of microorganisms — bacteria, fungi, and yeasts. It can also be the result of hypersensitivity diseases, foreign bodies, hypothyroidism, autoimmune diseases, disorders of the skin that involve its protective layer (keratin), other systemic diseases, parasites, conformation of the ear and ear canal, and even the use of inappropriate treatments or irritating cleansers in the ear. In people, food allergies and secondary cigarette smoke have been linked to ear infections.

If your dog has an external ear infection, he may shake his head, cry, and scratch the affected ear(s). The ear(s) may feel hot and show evidence of scratching and irritation. Gently swabbing the ear canal with a large chunk of cotton may reveal a gooey brown to black discharge.

Otitis externa responds to herbal and other alternative treatments. However, otitis media and otitis interna — infections of the

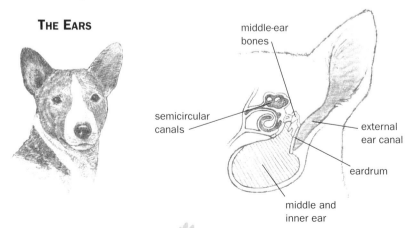

THE EARS

middle-ear bones

semicircular canals

external ear canal

eardrum

middle and inner ear

middle and inner ear, respectively — are problems for your veterinarian only. Be sure to get an accurate diagnosis before you begin home treatment on your own.

How to Treat It

In Western medicine solutions, the ear canal is flushed and cleaned, often under general anesthesia. Then various antibiotic or combined antibiotic/steroid preparations are used. Surgery to open up the ear canal to allow for better circulation may ultimately be indicated for dogs that don't respond to normal treatments.

In my opinion, alternative medicine is much better suited to treating ear infections. Herbs are a primary line of defense and my first treatment choice. I have found herbal remedies much more effective than anything I used from my Western medicine repertory for ear problems. In addition, chiropractic care of the neck should *always* be considered. Acupuncture and homeopathy are often highly effective as well.

In this chapter I present my own special ear treatment protocol.

Antibiotic and Steroid Therapy

Unfortunately, many of the proprietary preparations used in Western medicine contain corticosteroids (cortisone); the theory is that they counteract inflammation and thus diminish pain and irritation. I almost never use them anymore. First of all, steroids retard the long-term healing process. But more important, their list of potential adverse side effects is enough to make anyone who can read hesitant to use them.

It has been my experience that many of the antibiotic preparations commonly used for otitis do a fair job on bacterial infections, but the decrease of bacteria is often followed by severe fungal or yeast overgrowth. When you disrupt the normal "good-guy" flora of the ear canal (or anywhere else in the body), other "bad-guy" bugs can flourish. It's almost as if the yeasts and fungi feast on the drugs used in Western medicine.

Step 1: Get an Accurate Diagnosis

You must see your veterinarian for this step. First, I rule out all possible secondary causes (see above). Then I visually examine the canal with an otoscope and take a swab to identify the primary bugs involved and the severity of the disease. I use this information to decide on the overall treatment regimen.

Step 2: Employ Chiropractic

Many dogs with chronic ear infections also have cervical (neck) subluxations (partial dislocations). Is this problem the cause or the effect of the ear disease? I don't know, but adjusting the upper cervical vertebra (and the way it "hooks" onto the skull) makes sense to me. And I've seen some dramatic cures for ear conditions with chiropractic and mild herbs alone.

Step 3: Use a Vinegar Solution

If the ears are relatively clean, a mild 1:1 mix of vinegar and water, applied into the ear canal, may be sufficient. You may also use an herbal preparation (see step 5 for suggestions) instead. How often you use the vinegar/water or herbal solution depends on the individual case; it ranges from once daily for a few weeks to once a week or so for several months, then once every month or so thereafter.

Note: A key to curing ear infections is getting the herbal mixture in contact with the offending bugs. Have your veterinarian show you how to properly apply vinegar or herbal solutions so that they reach deep into the ear canal. And remember: As always, it's much easier to prevent infection than it is to cure it. I recommend using a mild herbal ear remedy once a month or so throughout your dog's life.

If you still aren't sure how to give ear medicines, have your vet or the veterinary assistant at your vet clinic show you how.

ADMINISTERING EAR MEDICATION

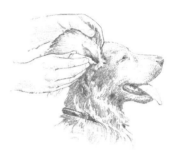

The key is to get plenty of the liquid down into the long, curved ear canal. Hold the ear up and away from the dog's head and pour (or squirt from a dropper) several drops (at least one dropperful) of medicine into the canal.

Massage gently below the ear.

Wipe off the excess fluid and any crud that has worked up from the canal.

Step 4: Add Herbs

For obviously infected cases, I use a variety of herbal remedies in a three-pronged approach:

1. When applied topically in the ear canal, the herbs bring the ear's flora back into balance.
2. When used topically and internally (as a tea, tincture, capsule, or tablet), the plants enhance the immune system and thwart microorganism overgrowth.
3. When used topically and internally (topically is usually more effective), the herbs relieve pain and inflammation.

Once again, how often and for how long you use the herbal mixtures depend on the individual case — from once or twice daily for a few weeks to once a week or so for several months.

Step 5: Other Alternative Treatments

For severe or chronic otitis, I add either homeopathic remedies or acupuncture. It's not often that I recommend any one product, but I have found Halo's Natural Herbal Ear Wash™ very effective for otitis — whether mild or severe, acute or chronic. This product contains chamomile extract, sage oil, clove oil, horehound extract, southernwood extract, calendula extract, pennyroyal oil, and St.-John's-wort oil in a witch hazel base. It seems to ease the pain in most cases, evaporates readily in the canal (leaving no oily mess), smells good, *and* is effective. This is my starter treatment for all ear problems, and I use it on my own critters as well for my human family's earaches. It is available in many health food and pet stores or by calling (800) 426-4256.

TAKING THE HERBAL APPROACH

The good news is that herbal remedies are effective against fungal and yeast as well as bacterial infections. So, herbal ear-infection remedies won't allow the yeast overgrowth common with antibiotic use. What's more, several of the following herbs (chamomile, mullein flowers, witch hazel) relieve the pain, inflammation, and irritation common with ear problems. This means that when using herbs, you almost never need to resort to ear medications that contain those nasty steroids.

On the other hand, herbal remedies are not a magic formula for all ear infections. Remember that herbs tend to act slowly. You and your dog may not be able to put up with the head-shaking, ear-flopping, whining routine while the infection heals. But it's been my experience that the herbal remedies actually work nearly as fast as other veterinary drugs, and whatever we lose in quickness of response we gain back with a more completely healed ear at the end of the therapy.

Finally, not all ear infections will respond to herbal remedies. In fact, I find the really chronic ear cases to be some of the most challenging problems I face in my alternative practice. Whenever I am presented with a chronic ear infection, I always, *always* bring out the big guns — chiropractic and either classical homeopathy or acupuncture — in addition to herbs.

The following is a list of my favorite herbs for otitis. Many of these are available commercially, usually as a mixture of several herbs prepared in tinctures or herbal oils. Look for them in health food stores or better pet stores. For an easy-to-make-at-home preparation for mild infections, see page 80.

Calendula (Calendula officinalis)

Calendula, which is sometimes called pot marigold but is not the same as the ornamental marigold you have on your porch, has amazing healing abilities. It is one of the best herbs for treating local skin infections and external ear problems. Used either internally or externally, it is a potent antifungal.

Chamomile (Anthemis nobilis *and* Matricaria recutita)

This herb is helpful when used both internally and topically in the ear canal. Chamomile's relaxing, anti-inflammatory, analgesic, sedative, and antiseptic qualities are the perfect combination for sore, infected ears. The herb also has a powerful ability to ease your dog and help him or her sleep through the pain.

Mullein (Verbascum thapsus)

An extract of mullein made in an olive-oil base (see recipe on page 80) is perhaps the best single remedy I've found for soothing and healing inflamed surfaces. For otitis, place several drops of the solution deep into the ear canal.

St.-John's-Wort (Hypericum perforatum)

Whether used internally or externally, St.-John's-wort has antibiotic properties. It's also a wonderful herb to calm the beast made savage by the irritation of infection.

Other Herbs

Some other herbs are also good for treating ear infections:
- Echinacea and Oregon grape root — when used together in a tea, tincture, capsule, or tablet — balance the immune system and help counterattack microbes from the inside out.
- Garlic *(Allium sativum)* is often added to herbal otic mixtures for its antibiotic properties.
- Witch hazel *(Hamamelis virginiana)* is an excellent astringent, decreasing swelling in the ear canal and thus easing pain.

Mullein Otic Mix

USE FOR: EXTERNAL EAR INFECTIONS

I like mullein as a home-brew ear medicine because it's so easy to come by: Simply scour the local fields in late summer and collect the flowering spikes.

Mullein flowers
Olive oil
Garlic

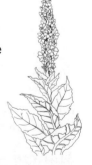

1. You can take the time to pick off the mullein flowers (a tedious process at best), or simply cut up the entire cob, flowers and all.
2. Pack the flowers or cob pieces loosely in a glass jar and cover them with olive oil. For increased antibiotic effectiveness, add a clove or two of garlic per pint of mullein oil.
3. Let the mixture sit for 2 to 3 weeks. Strain and bottle it again.

Mullein

4. To use, apply several drops of the oil (warmed to body or room temperature) to the ear canal. When stored in the refrigerator, the oil will last for several months.

Homeopathy and Acupuncture for Otitis Externa

I've found both acupuncture and homeopathy to be excellent therapy for otitis externa, and I often resort to one or the other (in addition to herbs and chiropractic) for a severe or chronic infection. However, these are not methods for an amateur.

It usually takes three to five initial acupuncture treatments before we will see good results, and for lasting effects we may need to repeat the treatments periodically. Furthermore, specific acupuncture application around the ear is a mite tricky (especially on a squirming dog), and a complete acupuncture treatment always includes other sites involved with immune function, organ systems related to the ear, *chi*, and *yin-yang* balance.

You probably won't be using acupuncture needles on your own pet, but for home application acu*pressure* can be very helpful. For this treatment, you don't really need to know all of the 300-plus acupuncture sites to help your dog. Simply massage the dog's legs, fore and hind, inside and out, from hip and shoulder — include the toes. Then massage along the sides of your dog's spine from head to tail; do this *gently*. Finally, massage all the way around the base of your dog's ears.

With this massage you've given mild stimulation to most of the important acupuncture points — exactly what I'd do, in a more powerful manner, with acupuncture needles.

When I use homeopathic remedies for any problem, I use classical homeopathy. The objective of classical homeopathy is to find the *one* remedy that matches the patient's constitution. Use that remedy appropriately and all diseases are cured.

I've had some miraculous cures using homeopathic remedies for anything from metabolic diseases to otitis. The problem with classical homeopathy for otitis is twofold. First, it may take a considerable amount of time to get to the correct, curative remedy; second, one of the last areas to heal is the ear. In both cases, your dog's otitis may linger longer than you (or she) would like.

The Eyes

The key symptom for eye disease is reddened eyes, often with a discharge that varies from clear tearing to a thicker, more mucuslike mess accumulating at the corners. In general, the greater the amount of discharge and the thicker and more gooey it is, the more serious the problem. Your dog may also squint, and he may refuse to go into brightly lit areas. Sneezing is sometimes a part of the overall symptoms.

Diagnosing the cause of the problem requires a veterinarian's thorough eye — and whole body — exam. Bacterial and viral infections of the eyes are common, and fungal infections can also cause problems. Allergies and air pollutants may cause your dog's eyes to redden and tear. Foreign bodies are a common finding, and since they typically hide behind the third eyelid, they can be a real challenge to detect. Trauma (scratches and pokes from sharp objects) can tear and ulcerate the cornea (outer coating of the eye). We need to watch these eye injuries closely to be certain they don't ulcerate further.

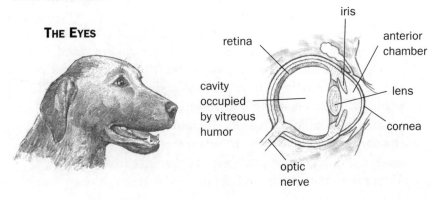

THE EYES

iris

retina

anterior chamber

cavity occupied by vitreous humor

lens

cornea

optic nerve

You also need to think about other problems that may be reflected in the eyes. For example, many generalized diseases, such as distemper, cause secondary ocular symptoms. Upper respiratory problems may make the eyes tear, and infections of the nose (rhinitis) may extend into the eyes and the sinuses surrounding them. Tumors can form in the eyes and surrounding tissues. And cataracts — whether caused by metabolic problems (diabetes, for example) orchanges accompanying aging — will cause gradual loss of sight and possibly tearing or redness.

Most of the eye problems I see in my practice respond very well to herbal therapy. In this chapter I discuss herbs that can be used internally and externally to treat a variety of eye diseases.

INTERNAL HERBS

Some herbs can be used internally to directly affect eye problems. Eyebright, for example, is used as an eye tonic. Ginkgo has been shown to be effective against diabetic retinopathy, and bilberry has been used to protect against age- and diabetes-related changes, such as macular degeneration, glaucoma, and cataracts. In addition, when used internally, these herbs have qualities that are secondarily helpful for eye conditions, such as anti-inflammatory, astringent, anticatarrhal, and nourishing activities. All of these herbs will alleviate the symptoms of eye problems while helping to resolve the cause.

Bilberry (Vaccinium myrtillus)

Rich in important nutrients that nourish the eye and enhance general visual function, bilberry also contains bioactive chemicals, called anthocyanidins, that help prevent damage to the structure of the eyes. Bilberry has been used to protect against both age- and diabetes-related changes, including macular degeneration, glaucoma, and cataracts.

Eyebright (Euphrasia officinalis)

An anti-inflammatory, astringent, and anticatarrhal, eyebright is an excellent remedy for easing discomfort and helping to prevent excessive tearing. This herb is rich in vitamins A and C, and it can be taken internally as a tonic for the eyes. It has also been used for centuries as an eyewash.

If the eye is infected, eyebright should be combined with antimicrobial herbs, such as echinacea (used internally) and Oregon grape root or goldenseal (both can be taken internally and/or used externally as eye drops).

Ginkgo (Ginkgo biloba)

Ginkgo contains bioflavonoids that are helpful for organs rich in connective tissue, such as the eyes. Ginkgo's antioxidant properties protect cells and their membranes and enhance cellular metabolism and blood circulation. Recent studies indicate that ginkgo may help protect against diabetic retinopathy.

Ginkgo

EXTERNAL HERBS (EYEWASHES)

Several herbs can be used as eyewashes. Many of these are antimicrobial as well as anti-inflammatory and soothing to the eyes. Although I have never observed problems when using any one of these herbs as an eyewash, some of them have caused allergic reactions in a small number of patients. Use them with caution and, for the first-time application, use a very mild infusion or tea.

Selecting a Treatment

My favorite eyewash herbs are goldenseal, Oregon grape root, calendula, and chamomile. Choose herbs from this list.

- Calendula: a potent vulnerary for wound healing, and a good antimicrobial that is active against bacteria, viruses, and fungi.
- Chamomile: an excellent anti-inflamatory and vulnerary that is effective against bacteria and fungi.
- Elder *(Sambucus nigra):* another vulnerary that is effective for inflamed and red eyes.
- Goldenseal or Oregon grape root: Both herbs contain berberine compounds that are active against bacteria, viruses, fungi, yeasts, and infections involving the mucous membranes.
- Meadowsweet *(Filipendula ulmaria):* a good anti-inflammatory and astringent that relieves red, inflamed eyes.
- Red clover: an anti-inflammatory for red, inflamed eyes.
- Self-heal *(Prunella vulgaris):* A weak infusion of this astringent herb can be used as a wash for tired or inflamed eyes.

What about Commercial Products?

Many commercial herbal eye-drop formulations can be found for humans and animals. Simply follow directions on the package — usually a dropperful, applied to the eyes three or four times a day.

Herbal Eye Compress

Some critters are more than a handful when you're trying to get drops into their eyes. If this is the case with your dog, try a compress — a clean cloth or a piece of sterile cotton soaked in herbal tea that can be applied to your dog's eyes for several minutes, several times daily. Always be very cautious when using warm liquids around your dog's eyes; the skin of the eyelid is thin and tender and can burn easily. Be sure to wash your hands both before and after the treatment.

> 1 teaspoon fresh or dried eyewash herb of choice, or a few
> drops of herbal extract
> 1 pint water

1. Simmer the herb in the water for 10 minutes. Allow the infusion to cool to a comfortable temperature.

2. Soak a clean cloth or piece of sterile cotton in the infusion. Wring out the cloth or cotton so that it doesn't drip.

3. Apply the warm, wet compress to the lid of the affected eye for 10 minutes, four to six times a day. If you use a piece of cotton, throw it away after use. If you use cloth, wash it separately in hot water with detergent and chlorine bleach (if possible) before using it again.

4. As an alternative, you can do what some of my clients do: Simply steep a tea bag of chamomile tea, allow it to cool to a comfortable temperature, then apply it over the eyes several times a day.

APPLYING AN EYE COMPRESS

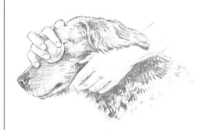

Place the warm, wet cloth or cotton directly over the lid of the affected eye.

The Gastrointestinal System

"It's not the germ, it's the soil," said Louis Pasteur. By this, Pasteur, author of the germ theory of disease and founder of microbiology, virology, and immunology, meant that the microorganism is not the major disease-causing problem; the problem is in the environment where the "bugs" grow. Nowhere is this more important than in the gastrointestinal (GI) system. I've found that nearly all the chronic diseases of a dog's stomach and gut can be corrected by paying attention to the GI environment. (See the "Acute Intestinal Diseases" box on page 88 for more information.)

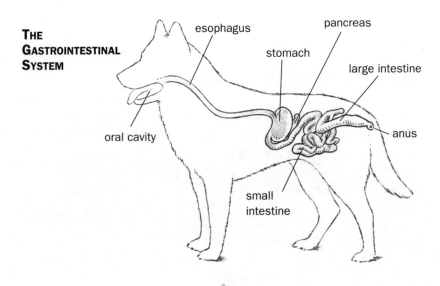

THE GASTROINTESTINAL SYSTEM

esophagus

pancreas

stomach

large intestine

oral cavity

anus

small intestine

86

We know that the billions and billions of microorganisms living in the normal gut are necessary to maintain a functional, healthy intestinal environment. If you alter this normal flora of the gut, you create problems. You can alter your pet's intestinal environment and change its normal flora by suddenly changing the dog's diet — giving foods he or she is not accustomed to or foods too rich in proteins or sugars. These sudden changes may cause transient diarrhea or even temporary vomiting.

The most common causes of chronic gastrointestinal disease that I see are those caused by indiscriminate use of antibiotics and steroids. (Whenever an animal is on antibiotics or steroids, I recommend concurrent addition of "good-guy" bugs, such as the *Lactobacillus* found in nonsweetened yogurt or in capsule form.) If you use either antibiotics or steroids too often or for too long, you set up a perfect environment for the "bad-guy" bugs to proliferate. The major bad guys are the yeasts.

HERBS FOR ACUTE GI PROBLEMS

I've found that the holistic answer to nearly all GI diseases is to improve the GI environment (Pasteur's soil) so the natural, healthy gastrointestinal flora can take over from the bad-guy bugs causing the problem. But I've also discovered that herbal therapy is often my best choice for chronic GI problems and for most acute problems.

Slippery Elm (Ulmus rubra)

For transient diarrhea *or* constipation, I've found nothing better than slippery elm. It is a soothing nutritive demulcent that coats sensitive or inflamed mucous membranes. It is the perfect remedy for the dog with an upset belly — for example, when a change in diet causes temporary GI upset. But this herb is good for any type of stomach upset. Give 1 teaspoonful of the powdered herb (mixed with water and given as a liquid with a dropper) per 20 pounds of body weight, four or five times a day.

Slippery elm is also good for the dog with GI upset due to tension or a change in his daily routine — the dog who will be in the show ring, for example, or going on a trip.

Slippery elm

Give the dose mentioned above several hours before your dog is to compete or travel, and then carry some along so you can repeat the dosage four or five times a day. Continue for several days, if necessary.

Acute Intestinal Diseases

Several acute GI problems may be life-threatening to dogs. Acute, serious diseases with gastrointestinal symptoms include parvovirus and distemper. If these diseases are not treated promptly, they may be fatal; you must consult your veterinarian rather than relying on herbs alone. When diarrhea contains reddish or blackish blood, or when it persists for more than a day or two, see your veterinarian.

Herbal Protocol for Chronic GI Problems

I see so many cases of chronic GI disease (referred to as chronic bowel disease, inflammatory bowel syndrome, leaky gut syndrome, and other, more colorful names not appropriate for a family-oriented book such as this one) that I think it will become the "designer disease" of the decade. What should we expect, after all, with all of the antibiotics and steroids used in a normal Western medicine practice?

My five-step holistic program for chronic GI problems is:

1. Soothe and heal the gut.
2. Reduce inflammation.
3. Reestablish normal flora.
4. Diminish the overabundance of yeasts.
5. Enhance the immune system.

Step 1: Soothe and Heal the Gut

My favorite soothing herb is slippery elm. For chronic gut problems, I might use it for 3 or 4 weeks initially, stop for a week, and repeat as necessary. Don't use it continuously, though; the herb is so effective as a coating agent that there is some concern it might prevent proper absorption of nutrients with prolonged use. Another demulcent herb for coating mucous membranes is marsh mallow root; use it as you would use slippery elm.

Step 2: Reduce Inflammation

Anti-inflammatory herbs include meadowsweet, wild yam, and licorice root. **Meadowsweet** is rich in natural aspirin-like substances that reduce swelling and pain, and it is also a diuretic and a liver-helper, thus aiding the body in cleansing and elimination. **Wild yam** is another excellent anti-inflammatory that has been used to soothe intestinal and arthritic diseases. It also aids function of the liver. **Licorice root** has a structure similar to that of the natural steroids of the body. It is an anti-inflammatory, used especially for gastritis and peptic ulcers.

Antioxidants are important to counter the excess production of free radicals. I use high levels of vitamins A and C, combined with antioxidant herbs such as oregano, basil, and thyme. I've also recently begun using glucosamine and methylsulphonylmethane (MSM) for their anti-inflammatory activity; they are especially indicated for the animal with concurrent arthritic symptoms.

Step 3: Reestablish Normal Flora

There are two keys to reestablishing normal flora in the gut: Increase the fiber in the gut and provide a healthy source of good-guy bugs. To achieve this, good-quality food is a must. Home cooked is best, but there are a few "gourmet" health foods on the market that have also worked well for many of us holistic vets.

- Supply extra fiber by adding cooked oatmeal, brown rice, or cooked wheat to your dog's food. Start with a teaspoon for every 10 to 20 pounds of dog and work up to at least a heaping tablespoonful per 20 pounds.
- Introduce good-guy bugs, including *Lactobacillus* and *Bifidobacterium,* by placing a dollop of nonsweetened yogurt atop your dog's food. Both are also available in capsules at most health food stores.

A third key for humans, but one we need not worry about for dogs (unless you sneak candy to FiFi under the table), is to eliminate all sugar in the diet. Yeasts love sugar.

Step 4: Diminish the Overabundance of Yeasts

For this step, I like goldenseal or Oregon grape root as an antimicrobial; each is effective against both bacteria and yeasts. These herbs are also astringents (easing the inflammation of the gut), and they aid liver function. Another natural remedy with specific activity against fungi and yeasts is the inner bark of the Pau d'arco tree (*Tabebuia* spp.; also called lapacho). This remedy has also been shown to have anticancer activity.

LEAKY GUT AND ALLERGIES

When yeasts are allowed to proliferate, they create a disease state that initially may be barely noticeable. The state is characterized by headache, lethargy, malaise, sore joints, low-grade fever, and other signs of allergic response, such as skin and ear problems. The most common cause of yeast overgrowth is an inappropriate use of antibiotics or cortisone products (cortisol-producing stress may also be a cause). These medicines knock out the good flora of the gut, creating a perfect environment for yeasts to grow in.

Yeasts are insidious in action, and as they continue to slowly grow and flourish, symptoms become more pronounced. Eventually, the yeasts' threadlike filaments (called mycelia) penetrate the gut wall to create a condition known as leaky gut syndrome. A leaky gut allows larger-than-normal particles of food and food wastes into the bloodstream — these particles instigate an allergic response that settles in the gut but ultimately extends into other tissues.

Symptoms of leaky gut syndrome include persistent and chronic, often intermittent, diarrhea that is sometimes blood-tinged or black from upper intestinal bleeding. Some dogs also vomit. Since the gut has initiated an allergic response, your dog will often have other signs of allergies: arthritis, ear infections, or skin problems.

With a leaky gut, you may get temporary remission of symptoms by changing to another dog food; however, the symptoms return when the dog has had enough time to develop an allergic response to the new food. As long as the yeasts are present and the gut is "leaky," your dog will eventually become allergic to any dog food you try, no matter what its hypoallergenic claims. Fix the gut, and your dog will ultimately be able to eat almost any food.

Step 5: Enhance the Immune System

Part and parcel of the chronic bowel syndrome is an immune system that has gone haywire. (Many of the animal cases of chronic bowel syndrome have a dramatic proliferation of lymphocytic tissue surrounding the gut — direct evidence that the immune system in the area is being stimulated abnormally.) Now, it's a good question whether this imbalance is a result of the ongoing gut disease or whether the disease process started with a compromised immune system. We'll probably never know. Whatever the case, however, in order to fix it we need to return the immune system to its normal functional state. Western medicine's answer to this is to use cortisone — temporarily reducing ongoing inflammation but in effect shutting down the animal's innate immune system for the long term. Good short-term results; perhaps disastrous long-term consequences.

In my mind, it's hard to beat echinacea in balancing the immune system. Echinacea increases lymphocyte production when that is indicated and reduces production when there are already enough lymphocytes.

OTHER GASTROINTESTINAL PROBLEMS

The following gastrointestinal problems are not listed under the acute or chronic problems, because they can be either acute or chronic.

Excess Gas (Flatulence)

I've known critters that seem always to have gas. (Come to think of it, I've been on long, exasperating car rides with some of those types.) And most animals will have a period of excess gas after their diet has changed. The same is true of the animal with a sluggish appetite or digestion: Some animals have occasional and periodic bouts of belly sluggishness; others seem always to be in need of a boost to their innards.

Carminatives help relax stomach muscles, increase peristalsis of the intestine, and reduce production of gas. There are plenty of aromatic herbs to choose from, and one of them should give you a whiff of success. Carminative herbs include:

- Aniseed
- Cardamom
- Cayenne
- Chamomile
- Coriander
- Fennel
- Ginger
- Peppermint
- Thyme

Any of these herbs can be the answer to your dog's aromatic activities. Use them as your dog's system seems to be asking for them to be used: If your dog is a chronic gasser, try one or more of the listed herbs mixed in with each meal. (Indian restaurants often have a small bowl of fennel seeds at the checkout counter, to help their clients digest their foods.) Try different herbs and different combinations until you get the correct anti-gas mix. If your dog has only occasional problems, then one or more of the above herbs can be used whenever you change from one food to another.

Sluggish Digestion

Occasionally dogs, especially older critters, will have a sluggish digestive system that simply needs to be kicked up a notch. My favorite digestion-aiding herbs include:

- Cayenne
- Dandelion root
- Ginger
- Turmeric

Since the liver is an important component of digestion, I typically add milk thistle seeds to the herbal recipe.

The same general instructions apply for these herbs as for the carminative herbs (above). Try one or more to encourage better digestion, whenever needed. Try different herbs and combinations until you find the one(s) that best suit your dog's individual needs. The nice part of all of the herbs discussed above (both the carminatives and the digestion aids) is that they are tonics and can be used for long periods of time, if necessary.

The Immune System

The immune system gives me the chance to discuss some important aspects of integrating herbs into a wellness protocol for your dog's healthy body and mind.

WHAT IS THE IMMUNE SYSTEM?

For starters, it's important to realize that the immune system is much more than just the white blood cells (WBCs) that circulate in the bloodstream. The WBCs (made up of lymphocytes and phagocytes), of course, are vital; they have the ability to recognize "foreign stuff" (everything from bacteria, viruses, and fungi to splinters,

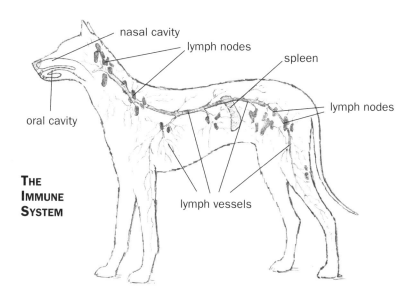

THE IMMUNE SYSTEM

dust, and the toxic by-products of diseases and body metabolism) and then to eat (phagocytize) that stuff and remove it from the body. But WBCs are not the whole immunity package.

The Role of Proteins

Also circulating in the blood is a whole army of immune-system proteins, including antibodies, the complement system, interferon, and interleukins. WBCs are not especially effective against viruses, but some of these proteins (especially interferon) are. Many of the immune-balancing herbs increase both the amount and the effectiveness of these proteins. And there's more.

How Other Organs Help

The WBCs circulating in the blood are actually a very small portion of the total number of these cells found in the body; one of the prime areas for WBCs is along the gastrointestinal tract (especially in lymphocyte-rich areas called Peyer's Patches). So herbs that help your dog's "belly" also aid his or her immune system.

The fact is, almost every organ gives a hand to your dog's immune system. The liver, for example, not only removes the toxins that decrease immune response but also is the prime manufacturing site for the immune proteins mentioned above. Add the thyroid, adrenals, spleen, and thymus to our list of immune-important organs, and it's easy to see that any time we help an organ system, we also aid the dog's immunity.

We also know that most of the cells of the body have a naturally protective, surface-immune capability. Cells of the lung, for example, produce a mucous layer that is antiseptic. Cells along the intestine produce substances (lysozymes) that are antibacterial and antiviral. Herbs that enhance individual cellular functions, therefore, also indirectly enhance the immune system in general.

TREATING THE IMMUNE SYSTEM SYNERGISTICALLY

Scientific studies show that a stressed or depressed mind lowers immune response. In contrast, a happy dog in a relaxed, loving environment probably has the healthiest immune system possible.

To summarize, since the immune system is actually an interconnecting whole-body network, I always use a mind-body approach whenever I prescribe herbs for *any and all* canine diseases. And since almost every disease, whether it is of the body or the mind, adversely affects the immune system, I remember to balance the immune system with appropriate herbs even as I'm treating another specific disease.

So where do you begin when treating your dog's immune system?

Step 1: Prevention Is the Best Medicine

Herbs are simply the very best way to keep all of your dog's body systems at maximum performance level. I especially like culinary herbs for this purpose, sprinkled on the food. Try oregano, thyme, turmeric, cumin, cayenne, and the occasional clove of fresh garlic for good measure. Food is medicine; medicine is food.

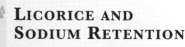

Oregano

Step 2: Create a Healing Environment

Healing should be both internal and external. I don't believe any medicine is complete by itself; to be effective, *all* medicines, herbal or otherwise, need to be "planted" in a healthy environment that includes good nutrition, proper exercise, minimum stress, low levels of toxins and pollutants, and frequent doses of hands-on loving care.

Step 3: Activate All Systems

Licorice root is my favorite adaptogen because it activates nearly all organ systems. This herb contains compounds with a chemical structure similar to the natural, anti-inflammatory steroids of the body. Its effects are also specific for bronchial and abdominal problems. Most pets like the taste of licorice root, making it ideal for use as a tincture or tea or as a flavoring to make other herbs more palatable.

As an alternative to licorice root, I may also consider one of the ginsengs (especially Siberian

LICORICE AND SODIUM RETENTION

There have been reports that sodium retention is a possible side effect of licorice. Use licorice with caution in pets with renal failure or those on heart medications. (See The Herbal Repertory, part 3, for more information.)

ginseng). However, I find that because most folks don't understand all of the actions of the various ginseng species, this group of herbs is one of the most abused today. I generally stick to licorice root, except in special cases.

Step 4: Activate Specific Organ Systems

Let's say that our diagnosis indicates liver involvement. For mild liver symptoms I'll include one of the liver tonics — turmeric or dandelion root — sprinkled as a dressing on top of the dog's food. If the liver symptoms are more severe, I might add milk thistle seed, either as an extract or sprinkled atop the food. And our old friend licorice root is also used in Chinese medicine as a liver detoxifier. Remember, by directly aiding the liver, we're both enhancing detoxification (see step 5) and indirectly affecting the immune system.

Your holistic vet will be able to tell you which organ systems require activation.

Step 5: Detoxification

All diseases produce toxic by-products that need to be removed, including dead cellular debris, dead and dying bacteria and viruses, oxidative and other abnormal by-products from damaged cells, and chemical toxins introduced into the body from a variety of sources.

My favorite "detox" herbs are burdock root and red clover. I like these two plants because they are well tolerated by most dogs; they counteract dry, scaly skin (a common site for immune diseases to manifest themselves); and, as a combination, they may have some antitumor effects. Use them in combination, preferably on your dog's food as a tea or sprinkle.

Step 6: Calm the Savage Beast

Nearly every animal I see in my practice is a nervous wreck, for one reason or another. If the dog is anxiously pacing and crying, worrying about being sick, I'll add valerian or St.-John's-wort to the herbal formula.

If Pet's compromised immune system has given him or her the nighttime itchy-scratchies, I'll offer

Oat

chamomile as a natural sleeping pill. I also like wild oat for its mildly calming, antidepressive effects. Try sprinkling these "mind herbs" on your pet's food, giving the dog the chance to select the ones that appeal to his or her inner senses.

> *S*ince echinacea does not simply stimulate the immune system but rather balances it, I am comfortable using it for immune diseases such as leukemia and lymphosarcoma complex, immune-mediated skin and gastrointestinal problems, and immune-mediated arthritis.

Step 7: Balance the Immune System

Our most notable herb for immune balancing is echinacea. Used on a periodic basis, this herb reinforces nearly all actions of immunity, including WBC production and activity and interferon and interleukin production. Echinacea also has strong wound-healing effects, is anti-inflammatory, has some antitumor activity, and is mildly active against some bacteria and viruses.

There are some minor differences between *Echinacea angustifolia* and *E. purpurea* in medicinal activity, but I use them interchangeably in practice. I use a tincture (nonalcoholic, if possible) of all plant parts (leaves, flowers, and roots). Since it has such a tangy taste, you may need to camouflage it — in a favorite treat, for example.

If you catch an infection early, you can often stop it in its tracks with low doses of echinacea, given several times a day (every 2 to 3 hours). For prevention and general immune-system care, I recommend a low-dose, on/off cycle; for example, 5 days on with 2 days off each week, or 3 weeks on and 1 week off. There is little, if any, scientific basis for this dosage schedule. In fact, recent clinical evidence indicates that long-term continuous therapy may be as good, if not better. But I simply have a gut feeling that an on/off cycle is more natural.

Step 8: Remove Invaders

The most common invaders are the "bugs" (microbes) — bacteria, fungi, and viruses. While herbs *can* be effective against bugs in the early stages, I try not to let any microbial infection get out of hand before I reach for a stronger medicine, even antibiotics if necessary. Echinacea, licorice root, and many of the culinary herbs (see The Herbal Repertory, part 3) have antimicrobial activity.

If you've caught the infection early enough, consider adding (depending on the location of the infection) herbs such as Oregon grape root for the urinary tract, calendula for the mouth and throat, or thyme *(Thymus vulgaris)* for the gastrointestinal and respiratory systems. Remember that, as a general rule, herbs are not as potent or as fast acting — nor do they have the same number of side effects — as antibiotics.

KEEP A HOLISTIC PERSPECTIVE

Your dog's immune system is an all-encompassing, interwoven complex spread throughout all organ systems, including the mind. Pet's immune capability is essential for health and disease control, no matter what disease we are talking about. Herbs are the perfect "medicine" to support the immune system at all levels.

DELIVERY METHODS FOR THE IMMUNE SYSTEM

Your dog's tongue and mouth may play a vital role in his or her immune response. According to recent evidence, when a whole herb first enters the mouth and touches the tongue, there is a whole-body response that activates many organ systems — particularly the immune system. In fact, this initial touch of the herb may be *the* critical part of whole-body response, especially when we are talking about the immune system.

So whenever we use the oral delivery method — sprinkling whole herbs atop a dog's food — we are taking advantage of all the orally induced responses. In addition, the whole-herb approach gives your dog the maximum benefit of the synergistic effects of the different biochemicals within the herbs, as well as the safety factors inherent in the bidirectionality actions of most herbs.

The Liver

The liver is the largest organ in your dog's body, and I argue that it is one of the most, if not *the* most, important of all organs. It is the primary site for filtering and detoxifying impurities in the blood. The liver processes most of your dog's food, converting nutrients and synthesizing proteins, and it manufactures bile that aids in the digestion of fats. Finally, it is a huge storage bin for several nutrients, such as glycogen (your dog's sugar source for quick energy), blood, vitamins, and iron.

Since the liver has so many diverse functions, the symptoms related to liver dysfunction seem unlimited. For example, many of your dog's gastrointestinal imbalances (such as diarrhea, constipation,

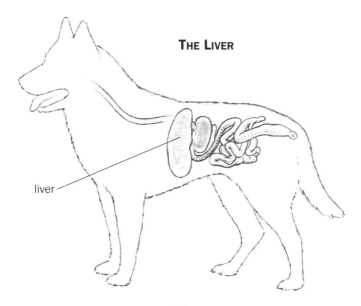

THE LIVER

liver

vomiting, bloating, bad breath, excess gas, and abnormal stools) may be related to liver problems.

Consider the liver whenever your dog seems to have a decrease in overall energy or has had a recent personality change — whether he or she is more anxious or more lethargic. Symptoms of the eyes (itchy, watery, swollen, red) and ears (itchy or draining infections) may be related to liver dysfunction, and your dog's arthritis may also be a result of liver imbalance. Finally, skin problems — especially acne and psoriasis but also rashes, dry and peeling skin, and slow-healing wounds — may be liver related.

Jaundice, a yellowing of the skin and the whites of the eyes, is an obvious indicator of liver dysfunction. Your veterinarian can analyze liver function by testing for liver enzymes in the blood. But I feel that many liver problems are already far advanced by the time jaundice appears or liver enzymes in the blood are abnormal.

HEALING PLANTS

Fortunately, a number of herbs are excellent for liver problems, and I've found that some of them are actually better than anything Western medicine has to offer. (If your dog has liver problems, you should read the box about liver dysfunction on page 104.)

What's more, herbs can be used no matter what caused the liver problem, because:

- Liver-specific herbs have several modes of action that are both liver protective and liver regenerative.
- Herbs typically have a broad-based sphere of activity, enhancing the function of many organ systems that, in turn, offer support to the liver.
- Unlike many drugs that stress or damage the liver as they are metabolized, liver herbs actually enhance liver function.

In this chapter I present my favorite liver-protecting and liver-enhancing herbs. Many of these herbs can be applied as a tonic for long-term protection for the liver — not a bad idea in today's toxin-laden, stress-producing environment.

Milk Thistle (Silybum marianum)

Milk thistle benefits the liver in at least four ways. It:

1. Is cholagogic, helping increase bile flow
2. Strengthens and stabilizes cell membranes — especially important for cells that have been exposed to toxins
3. Acts as a potent antioxidant and slows the inflammatory response, helping prevent further damage to liver cells
4. Stimulates protein synthesis, rebuilding cells that have been damaged from any type of liver disease

While all parts of the plant are edible, the seeds are thought to contain the highest concentration of medicinal properties.

I use milk thistle to support my overall protocol for healing whenever I suspect diseases of any kind in the liver or gallbladder; these include infectious (bacterial, viral, fungal), parasitic, toxin-produced, and oncogenic (cancerous) diseases. I've also found the herb helpful for other problems secondarily related to liver dysfunction, such as gastrointestinal upset, skin conditions, blood-clotting disorders, and dysfunctions related to the immune or hormonal systems.

Milk thistle

WESTERN MEDICINE AND THE LIVER

Despite the vital importance of the liver in overall health and well-being, in our culture the liver tends to be the most ignored of all of our dog's organ systems. What's more, Western medicine has few answers for liver problems. I get more questions from Western-trained veterinarians about the liver than about any other problem. Typically, their question is, "Doc, is there anything else I can do, from your holistic perspective, for this critter's liver?"

Truth be told, in veterinary school we weren't given much to work with for any disease process, unless the disease was related to "bugs" we could zap with antibiotics. Only through studying and working with alternative methods have holistic practitioners learned "newer" methods of liver care that include nutrition, exercise, toxin and stress elimination, body-balancing medicines (acupuncture, chiropractic, and homeopathy), and herbal therapies.

In addition, since milk thistle seeds are extremely safe to use and are readily accepted in food by almost all pets, I recommend them as a general tonic; add a pinch of seeds to your dog's food a couple of times a week. Active ingredients of the seeds are not very soluble in water, so teas are probably less effective. For the liver-sick dog, use tinctures or capsules/tablets.

Artichoke (Cynara scolymus)

Milk thistle may seem to be the cure-all for liver problems, but artichoke is yet another herb with similar, if not equal, application to liver diseases. And yes, Virginia, this is the same artichoke you relish at dinnertime. The only difference is that for liver protection, we use the leaves rather than the fruits.

Artichoke's actions are pretty much the same as milk thistle's in all respects, with perhaps a bit more cholesterol protective action (which is more important in human patients than in dogs). So use artichoke whenever your dog has a primary or secondary liver problem, and consider adding some artichoke leaf sprinkles to your healthy dog's food several times a week as a general liver tonic. Artichoke may also be combined with milk thistle — there is likely a synergistic effect when the two are used together.

Artichoke

Turmeric (Curcuma longa)

I usually think of turmeric and other culinary herbs as an adjunct to the medicinal herbs, but this is perhaps a mistake. After all, turmeric is an excellent cholagogue, and it exhibits liver-protective qualities similar to those of milk thistle and artichoke.

In addition to its liver-helping effects, turmeric also has:

- Anticancer properties
- Anti-inflammatory properties
- Antimicrobial characteristics
- Cardiovascular system benefits (inhibits platelet aggregation and interferes with intestinal cholesterol uptake)
- Intestinal benefits (decreases gas formation)

Turmeric is the perfect herb to sprinkle on your dog's food — I am continually surprised by the number of animals that relish its taste, either by itself or as a part of the mix of herbs called curry (usually a combination of turmeric, coriander, cumin, garlic, cayenne, fennel, fenugreek, anise, nutmeg, mace, cinnamon, cloves, black pepper, cardamom, ginger, and onion). Furthermore, nearly all the curry herbs are also helpful for the liver and other organ systems. Remember to purchase high-quality fresh or dried turmeric from a reputable herb supplier.

A Cornucopia of Herbs

There are many liver-enhancing herbs that I haven't used extensively in my practice, so I can't report on their effectiveness or palatability with animal patients. You may wish to research these plants further and discuss them with your holistic veterinarian.

- Astragalus *(Astragalus membranaceus)*
- Balmony *(Chelone glabra)*
- Black root *(Veronicastrum virginicum)*
- Blue flag *(Iris versicolor)*
- Boldo *(Peumus boldus)*
- Celandine *(Chelidonium majus)*
- Fringetree bark *(Chionanthus virginicus)*
- Schisandra *(Schisandra chinensis)*
- Vervain *(Verbena officinalis)*
- Wahoo *(Euonymus atropurpurea)*
- Wild yam *(Dioscorea villosa)*
- Yellow dock *(Rumex crispus)*

Other Herbs

There are some other herbs I often include in my dog patients' liver-healer preparations, especially if they are indicated for their other qualities.

Licorice. I include this herb in most of my herbal formulations for its adaptogenic qualities (which help many organ systems) as well as its anti-inflammatory and antistress aspects. Because of its sweet taste, it is readily accepted by most pets. Licorice is also an antioxidant herb and helps relieve intestinal irritations, especially ulcers.

Yarrow is useful as a mild tonic and bitter that helps increase bile flow. In addition, yarrow has anti-inflammatory and antimicrobial qualities.

Dandelion. In addition to its kidney-supportive actions, dandelion also increases bile flow and has mild antimicrobial effects.

Berberine-containing herbs. Berberine compounds are effective antifungals, antibacterials, and immune enhancers (by activating macrophages). In addition, they enhance all normal digestive secretions. This category of herbs includes barberry (*Berberis* spp.) and Oregon grape root.

A Protocol for Liver Dysfunction

Whenever I suspect liver problems, I recommend a five-step liver-healing and liver-protective protocol:

1. Decrease your pet's exposure to any toxins or agents, microbial or otherwise, that compromise liver function.
2. Provide food that has high nutritive value; low fat content; no sweeteners; and no synthetic preservatives, food colors, or artificial flavorings.
3. Since the gut is a common area that creates stress for the liver (as in toxic bowel or leaky gut syndrome), get the gut back to normal function by resupplying beneficial organisms (lactobacilli and other normal gut flora) in the food. One teaspoon to several tablespoons (depending on the size of the dog) of nonsweetened yogurt is a good addition to your dog's daily dinner dish. You'll also need to increase fiber intake — to decrease food transit time and provide a healthy environment for the growth of beneficial organisms — and decrease intestinal permeability via beneficial organisms and elimination of intestinal yeast. Don't forget to address intestinal yeast, or candidiasis (especially if there's a history of antibiotic or cortisone use or undue stress), and intestinal parasites, if applicable.
4. Add liver-protecting agents to the diet, including B vitamins, vitamins C and E, lipoic acid, catechin, cysteine, and lipotrophic factors (methionine, choline, vitamin B_6, betaine, and folic acid).
5. Add liver-protective herbs, such as the ones mentioned in this chapter.

The Nervous System

Like humans, dogs can exhibit a whole spectrum of nervousness, emotional stress, inner tensions, anxiety, and terror. There are dogs you couldn't rouse with a marching band; they are so calm, they make a cucumber look nervous. Some dogs are nervous Nellies, anxiously pacing the floor, yapping and whining at anything new in their environment. Others are terrified of almost everything: a car ride, the vacuum cleaner, or strange noises — especially loud noises such as thunder. Many dogs will go berserk whenever their humans leave them, incessantly barking and whining, gnawing on anything in sight, leaving a torn-up mess behind. (This phenomenon is so common in dogs, we've given it a veterinary term, "separation anxiety.") And there are dogs that are serene on the outside, but their innards are aboil with stress, anxiety, and nervous tension.

THE NERVOUS SYSTEM

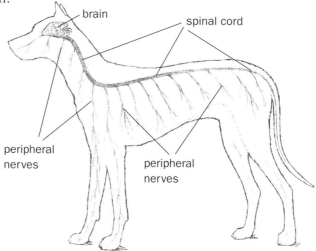

brain

spinal cord

peripheral nerves

peripheral nerves

HERBAL CALMERS

I've found that herbs are the ideal calmers because they are mild in their activity. Using the herbs won't make your dog "crash," as more potent tranquilizers do. The activity of herbs is short-lived. Animals won't wake up with a "hangover," stumbling around like they are in another world for hours at a time.

THE KIDD'S PET SERENITY SCALE

Individual dogs — and I suppose this depends on their own inner angels and demons, but who knows — have completely different rankings on what I call the serenity scale. Each dog has its own way of being calm and "in control of its emotions"; each also seems to have a different reason to go off the scale into pitiful fits of whining, crying, and cowering under the bed.

For example, Rufus, our golden retriever, loves to ride in the car — anywhere, anytime, for as long as we want to travel. He simply watches out the window until he's tired, then he curls up and sleeps. On the other hand, one of the most frequent questions I'm asked by clients is: "Is there anything, *anything* I can use to calm this savage beast when we travel?" Many dogs simply hate a car trip of any kind, and they will salivate, pace back and forth, pant, and bark or whine the entire trip.

Rufus is fearless . . . except in the face of two things: thunderstorms and firecrackers. At the first flash of lightning or the hint of a minor Fourth of July celebration, Rufus wants to be one of two places: firmly against my legs with his face in my lap or curled up under the safety of our bed. When I was practicing Western medicine, July 4th was a very good time for selling tranquilizers. Now I recommend a combination of herbs and Bach Flower Remedies, such as Rescue Remedy and Aspen.

Rufus loves all people and other animals, and he accepts being alone in the house without a fuss. Other dogs are agitated or just plain scared when other animals or people come around, and many dogs simply cannot stand the thought of being left alone in the house.

The bottom line is: When it comes to serenity (and its opposites, fear and anxiety), each critter has his or her own natural level. I've found that herbs can help create a calmer, more serene dog, no matter what his or her innermost fears.

While this is not a known problem with animals, it also makes me feel good that herbal calmers are not addictive. There is no cumulative effect — meaning that the herbs don't stay in the body and create a residue of activity from previous doses. In addition, some of the herbal calmers, particularly oat, are tonics; they offer overall balance to the nervous system. Since animals have been rolling around in herbs for eons, I feel that their systems are better adapted to the activity of plants, making herbs a much more natural way to balance nervous imbalances.

Remember to try these herbs *before* you need them to get a feel for your dog's individual reaction to them and the proper dose for each pet. Also, and perhaps most important, when Pet needs one of the herbs, take the same herb yourself. When you are calm and relaxed, your dog will follow suit. Just be sure to consult your physician or herbalist before taking a new herb, especially if you are already taking medication.

Following are my favorite herbs for the "serenity-challenged" dog.

Oat (Avena sativa)

This is the first herb that I consider, not because it is such a powerful antidote to nervous jitters but, rather, because it is such a good general nervine and so easy to give to a pet. Oats are used to strengthen and provide overall support for the nervous system. A pet with upset nerves can benefit from a daily or few-times-a-week dose of oats.

Cooked oatmeal added to your dog's food will help the nerves as well as provide a source of fiber. You can also grow oat grass (in a flowerpot inside during the winter). When it's a few inches tall, clip and serve (or just let your dog graze on the grass, as our critters love to do). Or you can make a tea from oat straw and soak your dog's food in it. If you choose to make a tea, be sure you are using organic oat straw.

Another way to reap the benefits of oats is to boil about a pound of shredded organic oat straw in 2 quarts of water and add this to your dog's bathwater. This makes a wonderfully calming and healing bath with high levels of skin-soothing salicylic acid. If none of these delivery systems suits your fancy, oat is available in pill and tincture form, or you can use the wild oat flower essence remedy.

St.-John's-Wort
(Hypericum perforatum)

This herb is terrific for anxiety and tension, but it can be used whenever your dog is depressed or needs some nerve healing. For separation anxiety, St.-John's-wort is my first choice, and I sometimes combine it with valerian.

Valerian (Valeriana officinalis)

Valerian is specifically used to reduce tension and anxiety, overexcitability, and hysterical states. Is it any wonder that this herb was a favorite of anxious Londoners during World War II? Although the plant smells like dirty socks, most pets love it as a sprinkle or tea atop their food. (Come to think of it, most dogs love the smell of dirty socks. Go figure.) Valerian is also available as a tincture or in capsules/tablets.

> ## USING FLOWER ESSENCE REMEDIES
>
> Bach's Rescue Remedy, Flower Essence Service's Five Flower Remedy, and other similar commercially available remedies are usually concentrated mixtures of cherry plum, clematis, impatiens, rock rose, and star of Bethlehem. Since the flower essence remedies were developed to deal with emotional disturbances, they are the premier treatments to consider for acute or severe anxiety, stress, and hysteria. They are extremely easy to give: Try administering a few drops orally by diluting several drops in ½ ounce or more of drinking water, or combine a few dropperfuls with several ounces of water and spritz (with a plant mister) the dog as you travel (or as Pet hides under the bed).

Chamomile (Anthemis nobilis and Matricaria recutita)

While Roman chamomile and German chamomile have slightly different medicinal qualities, in general they both treat anxiety in the same manner. Chamomile is a potent sedative used to reduce anxiety in a stressed animal. It has the added advantages of calming your dog's belly and helping her go to sleep. Chamomile, then, is an herb to consider before the car ride over the river and through the woods to grandfather's house — it will ease an upset stomach and may put your dog to sleep for the duration of the trip.

Some pets enjoy chamomile tea straight as much as we humans do. Alternatively, you can soak a small treat in the tea. Chamomile is also available in capsules/tablets and in tinctures.

Kava Kava (Piper methysticum)

A traditional herb used in Polynesian ceremonies, kava kava reduces anxiety, relaxes tension (including muscle tension), and calms restlessness — without a loss of mental sharpness or the kinesthetic senses (strength and balance) of the muscles. Kava kava is my herb of choice for a tense dog, such as one that is getting ready for competition, or for a nervous animal about to get a chiropractic adjustment. Kava kava is available in capsule, tincture, ground, and powdered forms. The ground and powdered forms can be made into a tea or sprinkled onto food. I've even seen kava kava in a honey paste — good-tasting stuff for us humans, but Rufus was not impressed.

Lavender (Lavandula *spp.*)

Another of my favorite calming herbs, lavender (*Lavandula* spp.), is used as a sedative. It's especially helpful to quiet the incessantly barking dog. Moisten your dog's food with lavender tea, or try the aromatherapy approach: Waft its fragrance into your pet's environment. You can even apply a few drops to the area behind the dog's ears. For a car trip, put a few drops of the essential oil on a cotton ball and hang it from the rearview mirror; you can also hang the scented cotton in the room that is your dog's favorite hiding place.

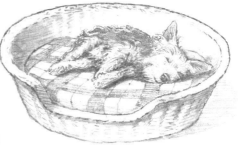

Your dog will rest easy after a dose of calming lavender.

Other Herbs

Others herbs to consider for the nervous system:

- **Catnip** *(Nepeta cataria)* has wondrous effects on cats, but it is calming to all critters. It's especially good for a nervous stomach.
- **Skullcap** *(Scutellaria laterifolia)* is especially good for nervous tension, and it has additional benefits for the epileptic patient.

Different Herbs for Different Dogs

For some strange reason (could it be because we are all individuals?), not all animals react in the same way to the same herb. This seems to be especially true of calming herbs and of painkilling herbs.

Using Rufus as my main example, I've noticed that he has almost no response to valerian, no matter what the problem. On the other hand, I have several canine clients who swear by valerian as the best thing they've tried whenever they need a calmer. And I've had other veterinarians tell me that valerian is one of the best medicines they have found for the persistently barking, kennel-boarded dog.

Rufus seems to respond most dramatically to chamomile; about ¼ cup of chamomile tea poured over his food will put him to bed within minutes. For traumatic events, such as the Fourth of July, I've had reasonable luck giving Rufus St.-John's-wort and Rescue Remedy, but he is still not completely at ease. This combo has had a full spectrum of results with clients who have tried it with their dogs: For some dogs it has miraculous results, for others it's as if they have not been given anything. And clients report all levels in between.

Rufus is much easier to chiropractically adjust after I've given him a dose of kava kava, and whenever I can get a client to give a dose of kava kava before a scheduled adjustment, his animal is also easier to adjust. I'm not sure Rufus is any more balanced or intelligent after a dose of kava kava, but he is certainly not any less able to run and chase balls.

The key is to try a variety of calming herbs, under the conditions when your dog is usually stressed, until you get the right one for his individual needs. You'll also need to experiment with dosage and frequency — each animal will have a slightly different way of internally assimilating the herb. The best part about herbal calmers is that your dog will relax *without* being "doped up" and "spaced out," as he or she is when taking Western-medicine sedatives.

The Reproductive System
(Neutered Dogs)

For several years now I've been recommending herbal support for neutered pets. Please don't misunderstand; I am not opposed to neutering. In fact, I don't know one responsible practitioner, holistic or otherwise, who doesn't agree that the benefits of neutering far outweigh the potential problems. We are all acutely aware that excess animal population is a huge concern, and neutering is the best way available for us to keep the population at bay. (See "The Number-One Killer of Pets in the United States" on page 113 for more information.)

THE MALE REPRODUCTIVE SYSTEM (NON-NEUTERED DOGS)

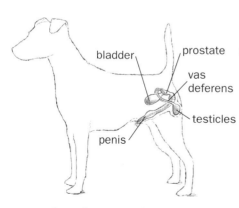

In male neutered dogs the testicles are removed.

THE FEMALE REPRODUCTIVE SYSTEM (NON-NEUTERED DOGS)

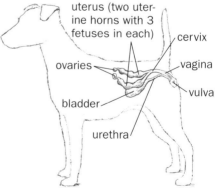

In female neutered dogs the ovaries and uterus are removed.

Neutering: The Operation

Neutering is a major surgical procedure performed under anesthesia and in sterile conditions. Since it is major surgery, there is some risk — both from the surgery itself and from the potential for adverse reaction to the anesthesia. However, when performed by an experienced and competent veterinarian, neutering is so low risk that we see an extremely low percentage of problems in the millions of animals neutered each year.

Female neutering, which is also known as spaying (from the old English *spayen,* which comes from the French *espeer,* meaning "to cut with a sword") or utero-oophorectomy (removal of the uterus and ovaries), involves an abdominal incision. Through this incision, both ovaries and uterine horns are removed to the level of the cervix. All female hormonal output from the ovaries is eliminated, as is any influence the uterus might have on whole-body systems. (See "The Advantages of Neutering Your Dog" on page 118.)

Since this surgery creates an opening into the abdominal cavity, several layers of sutures are used to close the incision. Depending on the technique and suture material used, the outside layer of sutures will be removed after 7 to 10 days.

Male neutering, or castration (although this term actually refers to the removal of the reproductive organs), also involves one or two incisions; this time, through the scrotum. After ligating (tying off) the vas deferens and the blood and nerve supplies to the testicles, the surgeon removes the testicles. Sutures may or may not need to be removed, depending on the technique used.

About Nuticals

A fantastic, recently introduced innovation of modern medical science has taken the world by storm — or something like that. Nuticals are false "testicles" made of synthetic material, and they come in a variety of sizes. Nuticals are meant to be used in place of the removed testicles so that the dog (and the dog's male owner) don't have that feeling of inferiority one inevitably gets when one walks around in public with an empty scrotum. This is the biggest bunch of silliness I've ever heard.

The Number-One Killer of Pets in the United States

Do you know what single entity in the United States kills more pets than anything else? The answer might surprise you. Euthanasia — the killing of unwanted pets by lethal injection or electrocution, better known by the euphamism "putting to sleep" — ends the lives of more dogs and cats in this country than does any disease.

Each year in humane organizations across the United States, millions of dogs and cats (estimates vary from 3 million to 10 million or more) are "put to sleep." These pets are commonly euthanized simply because they are no longer wanted or because they have a behavioral problem; most pets are not euthanized because they have an incurable disease. Even worse, no one knows how many more animals are euthanized by veterinarians or other individuals.

Since neutering removes the reproductive organs completely, it is the most effective population-control mechanism available. Over the years, other supposedly better or less expensive methods have been tried (such as intrauterine devices, injectable chemical sterilization, tubal ligations, and injectable and oral contraceptives). But so far the disadvantages — adverse side effects, difficulty of application, low levels of client interest, and the real inability to greatly reduce the cost of sterilization — have far outweighed the hoped-for advantages.

Occasionally I have a client who wants to know about tubal ligation (a surgical tie of the oviduct) for the female or vasectomy (ligation of the vas deferens) for the male pet. The problem with these procedures is that they leave the hormone producers in the body, and we typically neuter Pet because we are interested in more than simple population control.

Female dogs are less demonstrative than their feline counterparts when it comes to showing the world they are in heat. But if you leave a dog's ovaries intact, as in a tubal ligation, she'll likely attract every male dog within a 4-mile radius, twice a year.

Vasectomized male pets, since their testicles are still in there doing their job, retain the urge to mate, roam, fight, and all the other stuff that comes with the testosterone territory.

Why Use Herbs?

To be honest, I don't know many practitioners who agree with my herbs-for-neutered-pets reasoning, and there really isn't much documented scientific evidence to support the use of herbs. But I can't help but feel that the sudden and complete loss of primary hormonal organs (testes or ovaries) has a major impact on the entire body, especially the organ systems we know to be responsive to the reproductive hormones (estrogen and testosterone).

When I use herbs, I see improvement of some of the problems related to neutering — urinary incontinence and obesity, for instance. Again, I don't have any hard-core documentation, only my clinical observations. So even though I'm out on an unscientific limb, I feel very comfortable recommending herbs for neutered pets because:

- The plants act as organ-system balancers — something I feel the body needs after a major source of hormones is removed.
- I think it's compassionate to resupply some of the hormones we have removed by altering.
- When used in low doses and as tonics, herbs have very little potential to do harm.
- Although I don't have lots of supporting data (only my own positive clinical impressions), I think I've seen some herbally responsive conditions improve.
- I find that many of the dogs' humans, if they can use herbs to help Pet through the trauma of neutering, feel better about the whole process — which may make it more likely that they will have their next dog neutered.

One Week Pre- and Postsurgery

No matter what the surgery, I like to use herbs to help the patient get through the procedure with a minimum of problems. For about a week pre- and postsurgery, I like to give the dog the immune-system balancer echinacea and the antimicrobial Oregon grape root. This is one time I use a therapeutic dose — in nonalcoholic

Goldenseal can be used in place of Oregon grape root if you can find an organically grown product. Please don't contribute to the precipitous decline of goldenseal in the wild by using unethically harvested plants.

tincture form, or as capsules/tablets with the dosage adjusted from the label instructions to correspond to the dog's weight. In addition, I recommend a mild tonic, such as nettle leaves, to activate all systems and supply calcium, vitamin C, and iron.

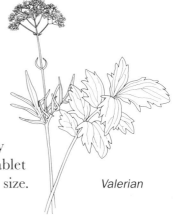

I think all animals become anxious when they leave the comfort of their own home, and especially when they are cooped up in a strange cage for a day or two before and after surgery. Valerian root and St.-John's-wort are great antianxiety herbs. Use them in tincture or capsule/tablet form, with the dosage adjusted to your dog's size.

Valerian

After Surgery

After surgery, I use herbs that might help body systems ordinarily influenced by the reproductive hormones. I also try to use herbs that help the whole body. It's especially important to support the following endocrine organs:

- **Adrenals.** Small amounts of reproductive hormones are produced in these glands, and supporting the adrenals, in theory, helps them produce needed amounts of hormones.
- **Thyroid.** My feeling is that the thyroid is almost always secondarily involved in any condition that is hormonally induced (in this case, lack of hormones is the problem).

Herbal Teas for Neutered Pets

I recommend a "hormonal" tea blend that includes equal parts of the selected herbs. Give your dog the tea once or twice each month throughout its lifetime. The foundation of our teas, whether Pet is male or female, always includes two herbs: licorice root and kelp or bladderwrack.

Licorice root works as an adaptogen; it supports all body systems. In addition, it is specific for the adrenal system.

Bladderwrack is my other herb of choice because, in my experience, hormonally responsive skin conditions in animals go hand-in-hand with an imbalance of thyroid hormones. Bladderwrack's thyroid-supportive properties are helpful.

To the licorice root and bladderwrack blend, I then select from the following herbs, depending on whether the dog is male or female and on other specific needs he or she may have.

SELECTING HERBS FOR FEMALE DOGS

Since we have abruptly removed the female dog's source of female hormones, we should serve her needs by resupplying some of these (or their precursors) in a mild and safe herbal form.

Wild Yam (Dioscorea villosa)

Wild yam root contains large amounts of plant steroids that are precursors in the synthesis of body steroids, such as estrogen and progesterone. Since their plant steroids have actions similar to those of other steroids in the animal body, yams have long been used for their beneficial effects when treating arthritis.

Dong Quai (Angelica sinensis)

Used as an aid for almost every ailment of the female system, dong quai also provides nutrients and helps tone the reproductive organs, making for an easier hormonal transition. Dong quai is excellent for the circulatory system, is a blood tonic, and is high in minerals, especially iron.

Wild Oat (Avena sativa)

This herb is used for its excellent calming and relaxing (nervine) properties as well as for its plant steroids, which may act as precursors of body steroids such as estrogen and progesterone. In addition, wild oat is rich in calcium and magnesium.

> *For the postsurgical male or female dog with anxiety, depression, or inability to sleep, consider using chamomile, wild oat, or valerian root.*

Nettle (Urtica dioica)

Good as a "booster" for dogs with chronic fatigue, nettle is a general tonic for imbalances in the liver, blood, nervous system, and glands. Nettle is also rich in calcium, iron, other minerals, and vitamins, making it an excellent herb for whole-body nourishment.

Chamomile (Anthemis nobilis *and* Matricaria recutita)

German and Roman chamomile are especially valuable for the neutered female dog that has problems resulting from stress, anxiety, and tension. The chamomiles are valuable because they are excellent, gentle sedatives that calm the dog and help her sleep peacefully.

Chaste Tree (Vitex agnus-castus)

Chaste tree is typically used in human females to normalize the reproductive tract at all stages of the ovarian cycle, including menopause. It is similarly helpful for dogs.

Ginseng

The ginsengs are among the best all-body tonics and are especially good for stress and fatigue. Although usually considered an herb for males, *Panax ginseng* may be helpful for the timid, cowering female who could use some added yang ("male" characteristics). Siberian ginseng *(Eleutherococcus senticosus)* is often considered the "female" ginseng. It is good for all systems, but especially the circulatory system.

Selecting Herbs for Male Dogs

Much as we can help the neutered (spayed) female dog, I think the neutered male can benefit from added herbal hormonal precursors. In addition to supporting parts of the body normally helped by male hormones (testosterone), we can offer direct support to the prostate.

Saw Palmetto (Serenoa repens)

Saw palmetto tones and strengthens the male reproductive system. It is an excellent herb for treating an enlarged prostate gland, but one of the beneficial side effects of castration in dogs is that the surgery greatly decreases the incidence of enlarged prostate. The herb also increases the tone of the bladder and nourishes the nervous system.

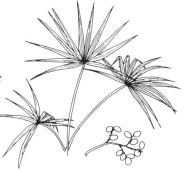

Saw palmetto

Damiana (Turnera diffusa)

This plant acts as a tonic for strengthening the nervous and hormonal systems. It also has antidepressant properties that make it good for postneutering anxiety and depression.

Ginseng

The ginsengs are particularly good for stress and fatigue. Most male dogs have more than enough yang (male) attributes, so only rarely is *Panax ginseng* indicated. However, Siberian ginseng *(Eleutherococcus senticosus)* is an excellent whole-body tonic that can be used for the neutered male dog.

Herbs for the Prostate

Intact (non-neutered) male dogs have a relatively high incidence of prostate problems, such as infections, benign swelling, and tumors. Although the incidence of these conditions is greatly decreased with castration, some males still have problems. Herbs that are good for prostatic swelling include saw palmetto, couchgrass *(Agropyron repens)*, corn silk *(Zea mays)*, and yarrow.

The Advantages of Neutering Your Dog

Without question, the greatest advantage of neutering is that it permanently and completely eliminates your dog's chance to reproduce. In addition, by removing all the reproductive organs and their hormonal impact, we have eliminated (or lessened) many of the secondary aspects of the hormones: heat cycles and all their trials and tribulations in females, and *some* of the roaming and aggression problems that are inherent in male dogs.

Neutering a dog at an early age also greatly decreases his or her chances for developing certain types of tumors associated with the reproductive organs, and, since they are removed, there is no chance for cancer to develop in those organs.

The Reproductive System
(Non-neutered Dogs)

I spend so much time and energy trying to get folks to neuter their pets (see the previous chapter and my comments below) that I sometimes forget that for some families, planned pet parenthood makes perfectly good sense — especially if they have already selected good homes for the future offspring.

Just because your dog hasn't been neutered doesn't mean you shouldn't maintain a holistic health-care system, complete with herbal therapies. Follow these steps to help a female or a male dog begin and rear a healthy family:

1. Offer nutritional support — good-quality organic foods with plenty of vitamins and minerals.
2. Create a loving environment in which the dog feels comfortable and relaxed enough to breed (the female dog also needs a comfortable environment in which to give birth and rear her offspring).
3. Enhance the dog's hormonal systems so they can express themselves in a normal fashion; herbal remedies are the natural, effective way to help an animal achieve whole-body hormonal balance.

For dogs with reproductive problems or other specific male or female diseases, I use a combination of chiropractic and acupuncture.

The results achieved with these two methods are often amazing. In addition, many reproductive problems respond favorably to homeopathic remedies. To support these therapies, I add herbal remedies and pay attention to the dog's diet and stress levels.

Neutering

Please neuter your dog. It's not just that we have pet overpopulation in this country; we can prevent nearly all cancers of the reproductive system by neutering. Neutering is one of the best steps you can take toward protecting your dog while reducing the number of unwanted pets.

HERBAL ENHANCERS FOR FEMALE DOGS

I like to use a cup of mild tea for the mother-to-be, poured over the food several times a week throughout the breeding years. Ideally, the tea should contain hormonal or specific sex-organ tonics (such as uterine and ovarian tonics) and a healthy abundance of vitamins and minerals. It should also enhance liver function (the liver is the site of production and metabolism of many of the body's hormones). For female dogs, choose two or more herbs from the following list.

Dong Quai Root (Angelica sinensis)

Dong quai is excellent for use over an extended period to strengthen and balance the uterus. Dong quai has no specific hormonal action; it helps regulate and balance hormonal production via its liver-cleansing and blood-nourishing activities. The plant is also a mild nervine, helping calm and relax nervous Nellies.

Wild Yam Root (Dioscorea villosa)

Wild yam contains steroidal precursors that have been used to provide the building blocks for a variety of steroidal drugs, including birth-control pills and cortisone. Long before its application in drug manufacturing, wild yam was used by herbalists to normalize hormone production; it helps regulate the ratio of progesterone to estrogen in the body. Wild yam is also a liver tonic, and it has anti-inflammatory activity.

Chaste Tree (Vitex agnus-castus)

If you read certain folklore claims about chaste tree, you might think its major activity is suppressing libido. But according to the French herbalist Cazin, the herb is sexually stimulating. The truth is, however, that chaste tree is neither stimulating nor suppressing. It is a normalizing herb that works through the pituitary gland to regulate female and male sex hormones. It is excellent for restoring and regulating the female's estrogen-progesterone balance. It has no known side effects, so it can be used for prolonged periods.

Chaste tree

Black Cohosh (Cimicifuga racemosa)

Black and blue cohosh are often used in combination for their synergistic effects. Black cohosh has an estrogen-like effect and is used to balance and regulate female hormones. During labor it may be used to aid uterine activity while relieving nervousness.

Blue Cohosh (Caulophyllum thalictroides)

Blue cohosh was used by Native American women during the later stages of pregnancy to ensure easy labor and childbirth. Today's herbalists consider it one of the best uterine stimulants available. It is also a potent antispasmodic that can relieve coughs, asthma, and arthritic pain. Since it may cause uterine contractions, it shouldn't be used in the early stages of pregnancy.

LIVER HELPERS

To enhance the production and metabolism of hormones, whether your dog is male or female, include one or more of the liver-helper herbs: milk thistle, dandelion, and turmeric. For more information on liver herbs, see chapter 14.

Nettle (Urtica dioica)

Nettle is valuable as both a food and a medicine. It is high in vitamins and minerals, especially calcium, iron, and vitamin C. An herbal medicine that strengthens and supports the entire body, nettle has a strong reputation as a pregnancy tonic, an antihemorrhagic during childbirth, and a therapy for a variety of female reproductive problems. It can also be used to enrich and increase milk flow and to restore and rebuild the mother's energy after birth.

Raspberry Leaf (Rubus idaeus)

Known to herbalists as the "herb supreme" for pregnant women, raspberry leaf has a long tradition of use during pregnancy to strengthen and tone uterine tissue. It's also used to assist in contractions and prevent hemorrhage during labor. Raspberry leaf contains high amounts of vitamins and minerals, especially calcium and iron. It is safe to use during all stages of pregnancy.

Mammary Cancers

Mammary cancers can be nasty in dogs. When there is a palpable growth in the mammary region, I recommend immediate surgical removal of the mass, along with a biopsy to help determine the dog's prognosis. After tumor removal, herbs may be helpful in preventing recurrence. I have tried some of the herbs with supposed anticancer activity, so far with varying amounts of success. Herbs to consider include echinacea, goldenseal, chaparral, noni juice, and aloe vera. (See chapter 8 for more information on herbs for cancer.)

Milk-Flow Enhancers

If your new mother dog needs a little help in getting the milk flowing, try one of these herbs:

- **Blessed thistle** *(Cnicus benedictus)*. The leaves of this plant enhance milk flow. However, the herb is also a digestion-enhancing bitter. Most dogs do not like the taste of bitters, so I usually stick to fennel and fenugreek for enhancing lactation.
- **Fennel** *(Foeniculum vulgare)*. The seeds of this plant are probably the best herb for increasing milk flow. They're also excellent for relieving colic and flatulence, and they've been used to treat coughs and bronchitis as well.
- **Fenugreek** *(Trigonella foenum-graecum)*. Another good herb for stimulating milk flow, the seeds of fenugreek are also used to ease sore throats and bronchitis. Externally, fenugreek treats sores and wounds.

Fenugreek

Herbs to Avoid during Pregnancy

Several herbs stimulate the uterus, and the resultant uterine contractions (which can be helpful during other times of the female cycle) can cause abortion. To prevent this, avoid giving your pregnant dog:

- Barberry
- Goldenseal
- Juniper *(Juniperus communis)*
- Male fern *(Dryopteris crassirhizoma)*
- Pennyroyal *(Mentha pulegium)*
- Pokeroot
- Rue *(Ruta graveolens)*
- Sage
- Southernwood
- Tansy
- Thuja
- Wormwood

HERBAL ENHANCERS FOR MALE DOGS

As with intact female dogs, non-neutered male dogs benefit from a cup of mild tea poured over the food several times a week throughout the breeding years. This tea should also include hormonal and specific sex-organ tonics. Enhancing liver function and providing vitamins and minerals are also goals of male herbal therapy. Here are some herbal helpers for the male dog.

> *Herbs can be the perfect aid to the reproductive system and the various stages of reproduction in both male and female dogs. I say this realizing full well that our canine companions in the United States are too efficient at reproduction — they don't usually need any help with the process.*

Damiana (Turnera diffusa)

Damiana has an ancient reputation as an aphrodisiac. Perhaps this is true, but, more important, the herb acts as a nervous tonic, an antidepressant, a urinary antiseptic, and a laxative. And it contains alkaloids that have testosterone-like action, apparently strengthening the male reproductive system.

Saw Palmetto (Serenoa repens)

Saw palmetto berries tone and strengthen the male reproductive system. They can be used safely when a boost of male sexual hormones is needed. Saw palmetto is also a specific herb that is used in cases of benign prostatic hyperplasia (BPH), a rather common finding in uncastrated male dogs.

Male Reproductive Problems

It's my observation that most male dogs don't need much help boosting their libido or their reproductive capacities. However, I do see the occasional dog with breeding reluctance and the rare dog with a diminished sperm count. Many of these dogs respond to better nutrition, added vitamin E and selenium, and tonic herbs in combination with mild herbal nervines to alleviate stress and anxiety. The initial nervine herbs I consider are wild oat, hop, and chamomile. In addition, try liver or general tonics, such as nettle, dandelion root, milk thistle, Siberian ginseng, and licorice root.

BPH in Dogs

Many intact male dogs experience a syndrome called benign prostatic hyperplasia (BPH), which is similar to the human condition of the same name. BPH is associated with an altered androgen/estrogen ratio and requires the presence of the testes. The preferred treatment is castration. I have successfully treated a few of these cases with saw palmetto, but I am always careful to make an accurate diagnosis; an enlarged prostate can also be caused by infection or a cancerous growth (adenocarcinoma). Infections often respond well to herbal medicines, but prostatic adenocarcinomas spread rapidly, have a poor prognosis, and, thus, require more invasive therapy.

The Respiratory System

With each contraction of the muscular diaphragm, your dog draws in raw air, with its nourishing oxygen, wonderful aromas, essences of local herbs . . . and all the area's pollutants.

The air first passes through an intricate labyrinth of mucus-lined tissues in your dog's nose, then travels down a long tube (trachea) and into smaller tubes (bronchi), and finally enters the microscopic chambers (alveoli) of the lungs. The air is processed within the alveoli; oxygen is picked up by the red blood cells coursing through the many blood vessels that line the alveoli, and carbon dioxide is passed outward to be eliminated during expiration.

All along the way, the inspired air passes through a maze of structures, many of which are coated with mucus and lined with

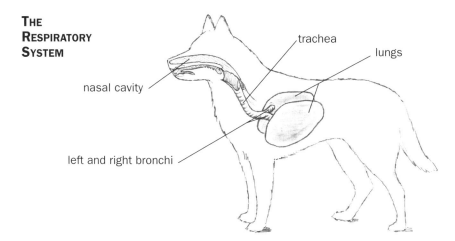

THE RESPIRATORY SYSTEM

trachea

lungs

nasal cavity

left and right bronchi

tiny hairs that constantly beat outward. These structures filter out the "bad-guy" stuff. At each step along its journey the inhaled air also experiences a complex system of immune-system checks and balances. The natural way for a dog to expel foreign material is to sneeze and cough, so a certain amount of these activities is a natural way to keep the system clean and healthy.

RESPIRATORY DISEASE

For a healthy dog, there's nothing better than a breath of fresh air; for a dog with respiratory-system disease, breathing may be almost impossible. Respiratory diseases can occur all along the system — from the nose (rhinitis) to the trachea (tracheitis) through the bronchi (bronchitis) and into the lungs (pneumonia).

Causes

Causes of respiratory disease run the gamut of possibilities: bacterial, viral, and fungal infections; worms and other parasites; cancers; and infiltration of pollutants. Lung parasites are rare in most areas of the United States, but they do occur. (The most common parasitic problem of dogs' lungs occurs when heartworm larvae are trapped in the lungs as they migrate from the heart through the body. These trapped larvae can create small foci of inflammation and pneumonia.) Cigarette tars are big pollutants. If you smoke, quit — if not for your own health, then for your dog's.

What Are the Symptoms?

Symptoms of disease in the respiratory system include:

- Difficulty breathing
- Excess coughing and sneezing
- Reluctance to exercise
- Shortness of breath

In extreme cases, your dog's gums or tongue may turn blue (from lack of oxygen) when he or she exercises too strenuously. A stethoscope will help your vet hear abnormalities, such as rough or raspy breathing patterns, fluid, or dead areas that indicate a total lack of air movement. As with any other health problem, professional diagnosis is critical.

Secondary Problems of the Lungs

When a dog comes to me with a persistent cough, the first thing I look for is heart disease; many dogs with heart disease have a chronic, nonproductive cough. Then I ask whether there are smokers in the house. Secondary smoke is as harmful to your dog as it is to you. Next, I consider the possibility of cancer. Primary lung tumors can occur, but more common are neoplasias (tumors) that have their origins in another organ and have subsequently spread to the lungs. X rays are indicated to rule out cancer.

If none of these problems is present, I almost always find that a chronic cough is due to a lack of balance in the dog's immune system. In these cases, I take a standard holistic approach to treatment.

THE HOLISTIC APPROACH

A good holistic protocol for treating respiratory disease starts with getting rid of irritants. Sometimes it's also necessary to use cough suppressants. Once irritated tissues are soothed, we can reestablish normal airflow through the lungs with good oxygen/carbon dioxide exchange into the bloodstream. Finally, the immune system is balanced, which helps stave off permanent damage from the disease.

Herbal medicines are a healthy addition to the arsenal I use to combat respiratory problems. I have found that acupuncture is often helpful for difficult cases, and I always evaluate animals chiropractically to be sure there is not a spinal or rib problem that may be hindering respiration. But many of the respiratory cases I see — both chronic and acute — respond very well to herbs alone.

Step 1: Eliminate Irritants

First, examine the general lifestyle of the people and animals in your household. Does anyone smoke? Do you use any chemicals for outdoor or indoor chores? What about special powders and sprays for gardening or cleaning? Exposure to any of these irritants can prompt respiratory problems in dogs. Foreign bodies that have found their way into the different parts of the respiratory tract are also culprits.

In addition to eliminating environmental irritants, antimicrobial herbs can be used to enhance the immune system's response. A combination of echinacea and goldenseal (or Oregon grape root) in a tea, tincture, or capsule/tablet is hard to beat. These herbs have mild antimicrobial activity, and echinacea is an immune-system stimulant. You can even add thyme for additional antimicrobial action.

Goldenseal

Step 2: Suppress Excess Coughing

Licorice root in tincture or tea form works well as a suppressant for coughs that seem to be located in the throat, larynx, or upper respiratory areas. Licorice root is also helpful for strengthening the respiratory system.

Mullein is good for deeper, dry coughs — typical of kennel cough or chronic recurring coughs that often begin as a bout of kennel cough (infectious tracheobronchitis, an inflammatory infection of the upper respiratory system). Mullein suppresses coughs and acts as a lung tonic. Use it as a tea, or put some fresh mullein in a cool-mist humidifier and let it run for several hours in the room where your dog normally sleeps (overnight is perfect). Smudging, or lighting a bundle of dried herb leaves and letting them burn so that the smoke permeates the room, is a traditional way to treat lung problems. Mullein can be used in this way; in fact, one of its common names, bullock's lungwort, comes from the traditional practice of smudging the herb to treat herds of cows with symptoms of autumnal pneumonia.

Thyme, in addition to having mild antimicrobial activity, helps relieve the spasms that are characteristic of coughs.

Osha root *(Ligusticum porteri)* is a traditional herb used by Native Americans in the southwestern United States to treat colds, flu, and other upper respiratory infections.

> **P**eople with decreased adrenal function are more susceptible to developing a chronic cough. This is probably true of dogs as well. Licorice root is specific for the adrenal glands.

Coltsfoot *(Tussilago farfara)* has a soothing effect. It acts as an expectorant, helping to move mucus out of the system. Also an anti-inflammatory, coltsfoot is a good herb to consider for either acute or chronic conditions.

Step 3: Soothe Irritated Tissues

Marsh mallow root *(Althaea officinalis)* and slippery elm bark are soothing to all mucous membranes, and they work well to ease a dry cough. Coltsfoot, thyme, osha, licorice, and nettle are all indicated for wet coughs. Turmeric has natural anti-inflammatory activity, and it strengthens immune function. As a natural diuretic, nettle helps dry out congested sinuses, and its hearty content of vitamins and minerals speeds healing.

Step 4: Reestablish Normal Flow

To reestablish normal flow through the lungs with good oxygen/carbon dioxide exchange into the bloodstream, try using these herbs:

Ginkgo has antiallergy and antiasthma activity. In addition, it relieves constriction of the bronchi.

Ephedra *(Ephedra sinica)* is a bronchodilator useful for asthma, bronchitis, and allergy problems related to the respiratory system. This herb is also known as ma huang in Chinese medicine. It attained recent notoriety when it was implicated in several human deaths. But the problem was that the preparation used was contaminated with the pharmaceutical version of ephedra and perhaps other drugs. This is simply one more case that supports my reluctance to use Chinese herbs — it is almost impossible to rely on their purity or quality.

If your dog suffers from respiratory problems, exercise may be difficult for him. Try herbal remedies to restore easy breathing.

Step 5: Balance the Immune System

Astragalus *(Astragalus membranaceus)* enhances the immune system and helps strengthen the lungs. Astragalus also stimulates the regeneration of bronchial cells.

Echinacea is my favorite immune-balancing herb. During acute bouts of coughing, I suggest therapeutic (i.e., heavy) doses of the herb, given orally as a tincture or capsule/tablet. For chronic coughs, I recommend the tincture or capsule/tablet form, used in an on-and-off schedule — 3 weeks on, 1 week of rest, then repeat the dose as indicated by your holistic vet.

Licorice root, along with supplemental pantothenic acid (readily available as calcium panthothenate or through foods such as brewer's yeast, liver, peanuts, mushrooms, soybeans, peas, oatmeal, and sunflower seeds), enhances the functioning of the adrenals, the master glands of the immune system.

The Skin

Iroutinely see three types of skin conditions in my practice: superficial scrapes, cuts, and abrasions; skin problems related to external parasites, such as fleas and mange mites; and chronic skin conditions from "who knows where."

The superficial nicks and cuts respond extremely well to herbal medications — so well, in fact, that I routinely recommend them in lieu of anything else. Skin problems related to parasites often respond well to herbal remedies once we have eliminated the parasite with a chemical treatment. (I do not find herbs especially effective against any type of parasite, external or internal.)

Chronic skin conditions from "who knows where" sometimes respond to herbs, but these problems are my biggest bugaboo. Chronic skin conditions top my list of daily frustrating cases, no matter which "magic medicine" I try. However, some of these

THE SKIN

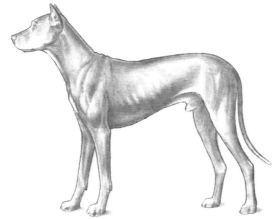

tough cases actually do respond well to herbs, so I continue to approach each individual case with hope and prayer — and a healthy arsenal of herbs, acupuncture, homeopathy, nutritional supplements, chiropractic adjustments, and whatever else I can think of.

HERBS FOR SUPERFICIAL SKIN LESIONS

Let's start with the easy-to-fix superficial skin lesions. There's a potpourri of herbs that can be used on minor cuts, scrapes, and open wounds. Commercial products incorporate one or more of these herbs into salves, ointments, unguents, oils, sprays, and so forth.

Liberally apply the salves, ointments, or oils to wounds that look like they could use some softening. Use natural-based products, and stay away from any product that contains an ingredient you can't pronounce. It is really easy to make your own skin remedies — often from weeds growing in your backyard or from easily grown plants. I highly recommend homemade products.

On a skin area that is red, inflamed, and oozing, use a liquid-based product that will help dry the area. I like to brew a tea of one or more healing herbs and spritz it directly onto the affected area several times a day. The tea can be kept in the refrigerator for a few days.

In this section I present my favorite topical skin herbs.

Calendula (Calendula officinalis)

Calendula contains the pain-relieving compound salicylic acid (also found in aspirin) and has anti-inflammatory, antiviral, antibacterial, and antifungal activity. Calendula also speeds wound

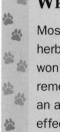

WHAT TO DO ABOUT LICKING

Most dogs try to lick off any medication applied topically. Since the herbs mentioned here can also be used internally, consuming them won't hurt your dog at all. (On commercial products, however, remember to read the label ingredients and be sure the herbs are in an all-natural base.) If your dog removes the external medication, the effectiveness is decreased. A pinch of cayenne added to each application of the ointment may help prevent licking, and cayenne is currently being studied for its anti-pain and wound-healing capabilities.

healing by enhancing epithelial tissue growth. In addition to having external uses, calendula is used internally for its antimicrobial effects as well as its ability to enhance liver function.

Aloe (Aloe vera)

Use the fresh juice of aloe for wounds, burns, and sunburn. Keep a plant in the house at all times so that you have a constant supply of fresh leaves. Then, when you need aloe's healing powers, simply break off a leaf and squeeze its juice onto the wound. Don't use it internally, since too much can act as a cathartic (laxative).

Chamomile (Anthemis nobilis *and* Matricaria recutita)

While its internal calming effects are well known, chamomile also seems to calm a pet's anxiety when it is used topically. Chamomile speeds wound healing and is especially good for inflamed lesions.

Other Herbs

Lavender (*Lavandula* spp.) aids healing, relieves anxiety, and eases aches and pains.

Mullein speeds healing and is soothing to inflamed areas.

Plantain (*Plantago* spp.) has gentle healing qualities. The leaf, used as a poultice, acts as a "drawing agent," helping to remove foreign bodies buried deep in wounds.

St.-John's-wort not only eases pain but also helps speed the healing of wounds, bruises, and mild burns.

Yarrow is an excellent healing herb. It also stops the bleeding from oozing wounds.

HERBS FOR PARASITE-RELATED PROBLEMS

The most common offender here is the lowly flea. Flea allergies account for a high percentage of the skin cases seen in most veterinary hospitals throughout the United States. The key, of course, is to eliminate the

The itching caused by fleas will make your dog scratch frequently.

flea. I haven't found an herb that is effective for this, so the main thrust of my herbal approach is to enhance the dog's immune system while helping the general health of the skin.

Echinacea (Echinacea *spp.*)

The primary herb for immune enhancement is echinacea. Whether using echinacea specifically for flea problems or for other conditions related to the immune system, I like to dose it in an on-off way: Use it daily for 3 weeks, then take 1 week off. Repeat as needed. Or use it for 5 days, then rest for 2 days. Repeat as needed.

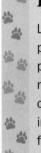

FLEAS AND THE IMMUNE SYSTEM

Look at the animals in any household, and typically you'll see one poor dog that carries the brunt of fleas. This dog is the itchy-scratchy pet and is often the one that also carries the majority of other sicknesses that hit the household. In other words, he or she has a deficient immune system. Some of these critters, if we give them proper immune-system balancing (see chapter 13), are able to shuck off flea infestations. And some animals can avoid fleas if their diet is improved with a bit of daily garlic and brewer's yeast.

HERBS FOR CHRONIC AND IATROGENIC SKIN CONDITIONS

Skin conditions can come from so many directions: bacterial or fungal infections; nutritional, hormonal, or immune-system imbalances; spinal nerve impingement; hereditary causes; and myriad other things that come under the heading of chronic ("we have absolutely no idea what causes this") conditions.

Another type of skin condition is referred to as iatrogenic, meaning "doctor caused." In truth, these diseases are usually caused by doctors using the medicines from their Western training. In other words, iatrogenic diseases are caused by the toxic effects of drugs.

With this in mind, it should be clear that a good diagnosis is imperative before you'll know which way to proceed with the herbs.

Find a veterinarian who goes beyond the quick fix of a cortisone shot and a flea collar. A good vet should give your dog a thorough dermatologic workup, including skin scrapings and cultures, blood tests, and biopsies when necessary. After the vet check, you can use herbs that support other therapeutic methods. Some herbs help create and maintain healthy skin and haircoats while we await the rare miracle.

There are as many herbs that aid skin ailments as there are factors that contribute to skin ailments. Here are some of my favorite skin herbs.

Burdock Root (Arctium lappa)

Burdock acts as a "blood cleanser," promoting excretion of wastes in the urine and sweat. It is a valuable remedy for skin conditions, especially those in which the skin is dry and scaly. Since some herbalists report a synergy between red clover and burdock, I usually combine the two in approximately equal portions.

Licorice Root (Glycyrrhiza glabra)

This herb finds its way into most of my herbal formulations because of its adaptogenic qualities; it is beneficial to all organ systems. And since most dogs like its taste, licorice is a good choice for camouflaging the bitter taste of other herbs. In addition, licorice root specifically aids the adrenal glands, which produce natural cortisone. Therefore, I use it for any condition for which I might once have used cortisone, and especially for skin conditions.

Sarsaparilla (Smilax *spp.*)

Sarsaparilla is especially good for diffuse systemic problems, such as chronic skin conditions. In addition, sarsaparilla is indicated for other chronic systemic conditions such as arthritis, and it has antibacterial actions for skin (and other) conditions caused by bacteria.

Yellow Dock (Rumex crispus)

Used extensively in the treatment of chronic skin problems, yellow dock, like burdock root, also benefits the liver. Yellow dock aids in the elimination of toxins that may be responsible for skin conditions.

Healing the Skin with Herbs

When it comes to treating skin conditions, I have a lot of not-so-happy memories. Yet I've had some dramatic allopathic successes. Then, when I shifted to holistic medicines, I began to see many more cases that, while they may not have been completely cured, got much better. And, of course, I see far fewer side effects than when I practiced Western medicine.

I remember Brandy, a 4-year-old Australian shepherd. Every summer Brandy was one whole-body mess of skin problems. When the temperature approached 80 degrees she itched, she scratched, she squirmed, she dug herself raw. Brandy had been to three veterinarians, one of them a skin specialist, and none of them had come up with a definitive reason for the itching. So Brandy had been on a variety of steroids, antihistamines, and whatever else the vet could think of.

I approached Brandy's problem holistically, without much initial concern for a definitive diagnosis. We changed her diet to a more healthy, home-cooked one; added vitamins A, C, and E; supplemented with other herbal antioxidants; and did a 3-week herbal liver "cleanse" using dandelion and milk thistle. For about a month we helped her immune system with echinacea and Oregon grape root, and we gave her some nervine herbs for the long term. Then we used licorice root for a few months and took her off all steroids, and I used the skin-specific herbs burdock and yellow dock.

In just 2 weeks Brandy's owner noticed that she seemed to feel better. In about a month, I saw her again and the changes in the skin were remarkable — no raw skin lesions, the haircoat had become lustrous again, hair was beginning to regrow in the bald patches, and Brandy was able to sit on the exam table without squirming.

It's been more than 3 years now, and once or twice a year we need to renew one or the other of the herbs for a month or so, just to counteract some early symptoms Brandy's caretaker notices. But other than that, Brandy's caretaker says the dog has had perfectly healthy skin since our original meeting.

Other Herbs

The combination of burdock root, yellow dock, and sarsaparilla (with red clover added for good measure) is my coalition of primary skin herbs. But since the skin is affected by so many other organ systems, we also need to consider those other systems in our holistic approach to skin problems.

For example, many of the skin cases I see occur in the "couch potato" dog. Lack of exercise makes for poor circulation and stagnant blood, both of which can cause unhealthy skin. Besides recommending daily exercise, I suggest **nettle,** which is a blood stimulator and has been used in people as a springtime tonic to clear chronic skin ailments.

The liver is also a critical organ for clearing internal toxins that may be causing skin irritation, so I might add a liver tonic, such as **dandelion** or **chicory** (*Cichorium* spp.), to my herbal remedy. If symptoms indicate that the liver may be a primary organ of concern, I'll add **milk thistle.**

It's my belief that all problems of the skin either initially or ultimately have an adverse effect on the immune system; herbs that rebalance immunity are always beneficial. **Echinacea** is my mainstay for helping the immune system, and it appears in nearly all of my skin remedies. If the skin condition is complicated by a bacterial infection, I add some of the antibacterial herbs, such as calendula and Oregon grape root.

Chicory

Finally, think about your dog and how difficult it must be for him or her to deal with the infernal itching and scratching. Some of the dogs I see have actually been driven crazy by the constant irritation. I think we need to do all we can to ease Pet's mental duress. Herbs I find helpful for the mind include:

- Chamomile, if the dog can't get any sleep
- Oat, for the dog who seems to need just a little calming
- St.-John's-wort, to alleviate irritability and anxiety, and for its healing and anti-pain characteristics
- Valerian, if your dog seems almost paranoid in her worry about the itching

Indicator Lawns

Many years ago I learned about lawn care and its impact on skin health after I'd been (unsuccessfully) treating a client's dogs for a recurrent allergic skin condition on their bellies, legs, and paws. The client also had a cat with early liver and kidney problems that I thought could benefit from dandelion root tea.

Thinking this would be a great time to demonstrate the power of backyard weeds, we walked out her back door so that I could show her how to harvest and use nature's medicines. After a lengthy search of her well-manicured lawn, and after finding not one weed, we checked the front yard. Again, nary a weed.

Then the light struck the dim abyss of my brain. "You have a lawn-care service, don't you?" I asked.

"Why, yes, we most certainly do," she answered, rather haughtily.

No weeds — none of nature's beautiful, healing plants. The culprit: heavy doses of pesticides and herbicides, toxic chemicals that may lead to allergic reactions — exactly like the skin problems this lady's dogs had been dealing with for years. Not surprisingly, the periodic nature of the skin irritations corresponded with the visits from the lawn service. When we got rid of the lawn service, the skin allergies disappeared, and my herb and acupuncture treatments looked like true miracles.

Ever since that eye-opener, I've made it a point to check my clients' lawns for weedy "indicator" plants, especially dandelion and plantain. They can tell me quite a bit about a dog's state of health.

The Thyroid

Every year I see more and more cases of both hypothyroidism (underproduction of thyroid hormone, a condition usually seen in dogs and horses) and hyperthyroidism (overproduction of thyroid hormone, a condition usually seen in cats).

ABOUT THE THYROID

For such a wee gland, the thyroid has a mighty big effect on Pet's entire body. Thyroxin, the hormone produced by a bean-sized chunk of thyroidal glandular tissue located along your dog's neck, energizes cellular reactions and increases oxygen consumption in the trillions of cells located in all parts of the body. So an imbalance of thyroid hormone produces myriad symptoms throughout the body.

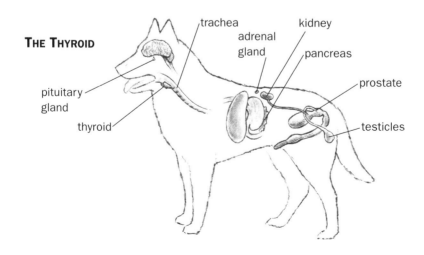

THE THYROID

trachea
adrenal gland
kidney
pancreas
prostate
pituitary gland
thyroid
testicles

Possible Causes of Hypothyroidism

While there is no simple, one-cause answer for the tremendous increase in thyroid diseases in dogs, the way our pets live in today's world has much to do with their thyroid problems. More than 95 percent of clinical cases of canine hypothyroidism result from the destruction of the thyroid gland itself, and most of this glandular destruction can be attributed to immune-mediated causes or other causes that are avoidable. Common causes of hypothyroidism are:

- **Genetics.** There is often a high incidence of thyroid disease occurring along a whole bloodline of pets.
- **Lack of exercise.** This decreases thyroxin output.
- **Nutritional factors.** For example, the thyroid requires iodine to function, but an excess of iodine can be toxic. Selenium is also a required mineral but, once again, too much can be toxic. Tyrosine is the necessary amino-acid building block for thyroxine. (See the box below.)
- **Stress or cortisol therapy.** Any source of cortisol decreases the amount of thyroxin available.
- **Toxins.** Exposure to toxic chemicals, pesticides, herbicides, preservatives in foods, heavy metals (especially mercury), and possibly excess vaccines (see the box on page 145) may lead to the autoimmune reactions that cause disease.

FOODS FOR HYPOTHYROIDISM

To help stimulate and support the thyroid, your dog's diet should contain small amounts of additional iodine, zinc, copper, and tyrosine.
- **Iodine** sources include sea vegetables, such as the seaweeds listed on page 143, and sea salt. Cod-liver oil also contains traces of iodine. *Note:* Many areas of our seas have been contaminated with heavy metals. For this reason, know the source of your sea herbs and salts.
- **Zinc** sources include beef, oatmeal, chicken, seafood, liver, dried beans, bran, spinach, seeds, and nuts.
- **Copper** can be found in liver and other organ meats, eggs, yeast, legumes, nuts, and raisins.
- **Tyrosine** (from phenylalanine, another amino acid) is found in soy products, beef, chicken, and fish.

Symptoms of Hypothyroidism

Although hypothyroidism can be seen in all animals, it is most common in middle-aged (4- to 10-year-old), mid- to large-sized dogs.

The symptoms of hypothyroidism include:

- Intolerance of cold temperatures
- Intolerance of exercise
- Lethargy
- Mental dullness
- Weight gain without a corresponding increase in appetite

In general appearance, the hypothyroid animal is ADR (Ain't Doin' Right). Skin and haircoat problems are common and include dryness, excessive shedding, retarded hair growth leading to thinning or actual loss of portions of the coat, and sometimes even a swelling — especially around the face — that gives the dog a classic "tragic look."

The typical dog I see with hypothyroidism has a sparse, thinning haircoat. The hair and skin are dry, and because the haircoat is so thin, it feels and looks much like puppy fur. Often the skin is discolored black, particularly under the armpits and along the inner flanks. Clients frequently complain that their dog doesn't seem to have as much energy as he once did and that he always seems cold, shivers, and wants to sleep right next to the heater or baseboard in wintertime.

Although you would expect a hypothyroid animal to gain weight, this has not always been the case with my patients. In fact, many of my hypothyroid animals are actually thinner than normal. Go figure.

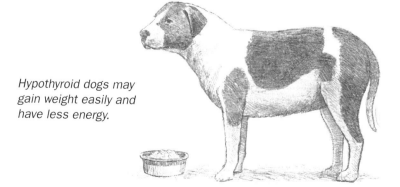

Hypothyroid dogs may gain weight easily and have less energy.

Diagnosing Hypothyroidism

What with the plethora of symptoms that *may* indicate thyroid disease, accurate diagnosis is difficult at best. The initial screening test for hypothyroidism, called the T-4 test, may show normal results when the thyroid function is actually decreased (hypothyroid). Conversely, T-4 is often low when other diseases, which are unrelated to the thyroid, are really the cause of the observed symptoms. Another diagnostic tool, the thyroid-stimulating hormone (TSH) test, adds to the accuracy of our thyroid-testing methods, but even this test is not always definitive.

The bottom line: If your dog is tested and the T-4 test result is low, wait at least 30 days. If possible, clear up any ongoing diseases, then have your vet redo the T-4. If the T-4 is still low, have a TSH test performed.

In the meantime, while you're waiting to determine whether your dog's thyroid actually is diseased, you can go ahead with herbal, nutritional, and detoxification therapy. If your dog's response is good (good response to therapy is a valid diagnostic tool), there's really no need to get uptight about test results.

ONE FINAL WORD ABOUT THYROID TESTS

I've had reasonable success treating both hyper- and hypothyroidism using alternative medicines only. But I have noticed that in some of the animals I am treating, even though their symptoms have disappeared — that is, by all external appearances they have returned to a normally functioning critter — their T-4 levels may remain abnormal for several months. I caution folks that we may need to wait at least several months before the blood tests return to normal.

Treating Thyroid Imbalances

In addition to herbs, the treatment of hypothyroidism should include proper nutrition, plenty of exercise, removal of possible causes of toxicity (including drugs), minimization of stress, and appropriate thyroid supplementation when indicated. Typically, I add acupuncture or classical homeopathy to the above protocol.

Conventional treatment for hypothyroidism involves supplementing the diet with a synthetic thyroxin in an attempt to come up with the dosage of the drug that supplies the amount of hormone that a normally functioning gland would provide. The problem with this approach is that because a supply of synthetic thyroid is readily available, the gland's feedback system tells it that it does not need to produce any more hormone. So the thyroid shuts down, and it may never again be able to function properly.

Although I've treated some cases of severe hypothyroidism in which it has eventually become necessary to add synthetic thyroid supplementation, for the most part I've been able to stimulate normal thyroid function with homeopathic levels of thyroxin, along with herbs and other therapies. With this approach, we are often able to safely return the thyroid to its normally functioning levels.

HERBS FOR HYPOTHYROIDISM

Herbs are the perfect adjunct for a holistic treatment for hypothyroidism. Remember that the last thing we want to do is to totally shut down the thyroid (with heavy doses of thyroid supplements); in fact, we want to do all we can to use whatever natural ability the thyroid has left. Bladderwrack (and the other seaweeds) is the ideal herb to help coax the thyroid to respond. Other herbs, such as licorice root and Siberian ginseng, are then used to enhance whole-body systems. And finally, we look at the dog's symptoms to see whether any other body systems could benefit from an herbal boost. We then use the herbs that apply to those systems.

Seaweeds

There are many types of seaweed herbs, the names of which are often used interchangeably, including:

- Arame *(Ecklonia bicyclis)*
- Bladderwrack *(Fucus vesiculosus)*
- Dulse *(Palmaria palmata)*
- Hijiki (also called hiziki)
- Irish moss *(Chondrus crispus)*
- Kelp (*Laminaria* spp.); often other species of seaweeds are simply called kelp
- Kombu (*Laminaria* spp.)
- Nori (*Porphyra* spp.)
- Wakame (*Undaria* spp.)

All of these sea herbs contain high levels of nutrient minerals and vitamins, and they are the best sources of plant iodine found anywhere. They are considered specific herbs for the underactive thyroid gland.

In addition, many seaweeds have other effects on the body. For example, bladderwrack is used to help treat rheumatism and rheumatoid arthritis. Thanks to its expectorant and demulcent actions, Irish moss may be used for respiratory problems such as bronchitis or as an aid for treating gastritis or ulcers. Kelp is used in Chinese medicine to soften hard lumps or tumors. The alginate found in many of the *Laminaria* species prevents the absorption of strontium 90, making them possible counters to heavy-metal poisoning.

Siberian Ginseng (Eleutherococcus senticosus)

A nonspecific herb for this condition, Siberian ginseng helps prevent both thyroid atrophy and hyperplasia. In addition, its adaptogenic qualities act to strengthen and balance all organ systems.

Licorice Root (Glycyrrhiza glabra)

Another nonspecific herb used for its adaptogenic qualities, licorice root strengthens and balances the whole body. Licorice root is also a specific herb for the adrenal glands, considered by some to be the master glands of the hormonal system.

Other Herbs

When treating hypothyroidism, I also try to think in terms of which organ systems seem to be the most adversely affected. For example, if the skin is showing severe signs of the disease, I would add skin-helper herbs, such as yellow dock, Oregon grape root, sarsaparilla, burdock, and licorice root. And since the liver is almost always involved in any disease, I usually include a liver-specific herb, such as milk thistle or dandelion root.

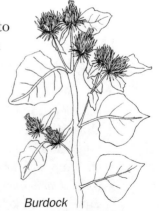

Burdock

CONSUMER ALERT

Heavy metals, especially mercury, can be toxic to the thyroid. Many of our vaccines are preserved with thimerosal, a combination of ethyl mercuric chloride, thiosalicylic acid, sodium hydroxide, and ethanol. (Vaccines may also contain a further litany of bad-guy stuff, including antibiotics, aluminum gels, formaldehyde, monosodium glutamate, egg proteins, and sulfites — each of which has been implicated in immune reactions in some individuals.)

According to a recently published warning from the ever-alert U.S. government, some human vaccines containing thimerosal, when given to infants, may produce internal levels of mercury that exceed recommended safety levels. Now, I don't know of any similar studies on thimerosal in animals, but I do know that many of our critter vaccines also contain thimerosal as a preservative. And I know that a 1-pound pup is a whole lot smaller than the normal-sized kid getting vaccinated.

Why are we seeing so many thyroid problems in our animals today? Perhaps one answer lies in the preservatives of our vaccines — possibly coupled with the stress we put on the animals' immune system. Thimerosal: one more good reason to question the practice of annual vaccines for Pet.

The Urinary System

There are two relatively common urinary-system diseases in dogs that respond well to herbal remedies: bladder infections (cystitis) and bladder stones (urolithiasis).

How to Diagnose a Urinary Disease

With a bladder infection or bladder stones, your dog may show almost the same symptoms. He may try to urinate more frequently and may strain during urination, and the urinary flow may be more of a dribble than a stream. You may see blood in the urine, although sometimes blood is evident only on a microscopic exam. Your dog may exhibit some pain when attempting to urinate, and some house-trained dogs may urinate in an inappropriate place — on the living room floor, for example, or on the couch.

THE URINARY SYSTEM

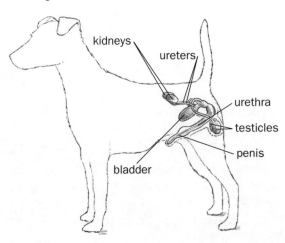

kidneys

ureters

urethra

testicles

penis

bladder

What to Do

First, take your dog to the veterinarian right away. The vet will do a urinalysis and perhaps take X rays, do a CBC, or perform other tests. Important findings from the urinalysis include specific gravity (measures the functional ability of the kidney tubules); pH (may indicate stones or infection); and the presence of blood (indicates loss of integrity to the wall of the bladder, urethra, ureters, or kidneys), white blood cells (an indication of infection), or crystals (indicating the possibility of bladder stones). The urinalysis and other tests help in determining a diagnosis and choosing the best treatment.

Correcting the Problem

Bacterial bladder infections are a fairly common finding, and I've had results with herbs that just about equal those I have had with allopathic drugs. Bladder stones are a different matter. Stones often require a holistic approach of nutritional change, herbs, and possibly homeopathy or acupuncture. Larger stones may require surgery, and recurrence remains a problem. Check with your holistic vet for the proper protocol.

TREATING WITH HERBS

With herbal therapy, we are trying to accomplish three major goals:

1. Increase urine flow. With this flushing action, we help eliminate the bacteria that cause ongoing infections, and we can prevent recurrence of infections. Because chronic bladder infections are a cause of stone formation, by diluting the urine we also decrease the formation of stones. And with a little luck, the increased urine flow may flush out smaller stones that have already formed.

2. Directly address any bladder infection. Some herbs have mild antibiotic activity, and many herbs help the animal's immune system deal with the invading organisms.

3. Coat the bladder and urethra with soothing herbs (urinary demulcents). Bladder irritation can cause nerve reaction that ultimately leads to spastic contraction of the urethral walls, resulting in pooling of the urine and, thus, a better environment for infection and stone formation.

The two herbal remedies I routinely start with for any chronic, recurring urinary problems are dandelion root and Oregon grape root.

Dandelion Root
(Taraxacum officinale)

This common weed is a potent diuretic, meaning it will make your dog urinate like a racehorse. I use dandelion for both bladder stones and infections. In addition to its diuretic action, dandelion root provides specific healing actions for the liver and gallbladder. It is also a wonderful general tonic. Since I believe that the bladder is often merely a repository for an animal's more general problems of the body, mind, and spirit, this is all the more reason for a general body tonic.

> *I*ncidentally, diuretics tend to cause a loss of potassium in the urine, and all animals can be very sensitive to loss of this important mineral. However, dandelion is an excellent source of potassium, so it naturally resupplies the loss.

Oregon Grape Root (Mahonia spp.)

Because we now recognize that goldenseal is a seriously threatened species, I have substituted Oregon grape root for the endangered herb — and I find it to be equally effective clinically. Oregon grape root's usefulness in fighting infections is due to its high level of berberine, a substance with strong antimicrobial qualities. In addition, the herb stimulates the flow of bile and, like dandelion, it has general tonic properties.

How to Use Dandelion and Oregon Grape

My best successes with these two herbs occur when we have caught an infectious disease in its very earliest stages. I recommend small oral doses of 1 to 3 drops of the (nonalcoholic, if possible) tincture of each herb, five or six times a day. Continue until your dog goes to the fire hydrant regularly, develops a normal flow (without straining), and produces good-sized puddles. You can then cut back from this therapeutic dose and go to a preventive/maintenance dose (see the next page). If your dog shows signs of recurrence of active infection, return to the above therapeutic dose.

For prevention or maintenance, use only the dandelion root long term. Give your dog one dose (several drops) of the tincture, or up to a teaspoon of the ground root sprinkled on the food a few days each week. Oregon grape root can be used on and off — for example, 1 week a month on and 3 weeks off — but long-term use of this plant (or any of the berberine-containing herbs) may decrease the normal, good-guy bacteria in the gut. Whenever you use Oregon grape root, add a teaspoonful or so of plain, unsweetened yogurt to your dog's dinner dish.

Other Herbs

There are some other herbs I consider using for urinary problems, depending on the specific condition.

Nettle, or stinging nettle, is a diuretic, astringent, and general tonic that is most useful for the animal that is experiencing painful urination. Nettle is also specific for respiratory allergies, and the root has recently been proved effective for benign prostatic enlargement (BPE); add it to the herbal formula of any pet with these conditions. Dried nettle leaves do not sting like the fresh leaves, and they can be used long term as a general tonic, sprinkled on your dog's food. The leaves or roots can also be made into a tea to moisten the food.

Cranberry *(Vaccinium macrocarpon)* acidifies the urine, which helps control bacteria, and it contains a substance that acts as a barrier to keep bacteria from attaching to the bladder wall. All this is great for bacterial infections, but the problem is getting your dog to drink something that tastes of cranberry.

Cranberry capsules are an answer for easy-to-pill critters, but most herbal capsules are large, so they're not practical for small dogs. You can, of course, break open the capsules and hide the contents in your dog's food, but I have not had much luck with this method. However, there are exceptions to every rule, so don't be deterred from trying cranberry on your dog. Remember, too, that most of the store-bought cranberry juices are sweetened and not appropriate for use; the sweetener will only make the urinary problem worse.

Cranberry

Herbs for Bleeding

Bloody urine is *not* something to fool around with; consult your vet immediately for an accurate diagnosis. After the vet has made a diagnosis and you are confident that you are on the right track therapeutically, there are some herbs you can use. Some act as astringents, which tighten connective tissue, helping to control bleeding; others are demulcents, which soothe irritated tissue and help prevent spastic contraction of the urethra, making it more comfortable for your dog to urinate when she needs to.

The following herbs can be used to help along other bladder infection or bladder stones therapies.

- **Astringents:** Horsetail *(Equisetum arvense)* and plantain *(Plantago major)*
- **Demulcents:** Corn silk *(Zea mays)* and marsh mallow leaf *(Althaea officinalis)*

 ABOUT UVA-URSI

Also known as bearberry, uva-ursi *(Arctostaphylos uva-ursi)* is an effective herb for urinary problems, both infections and stones. However, its effectiveness is limited to alkaline urine, and since meat eaters typically have acidic urine, it is usually not appropriate for dogs.

part 3

The Herbal Repertory

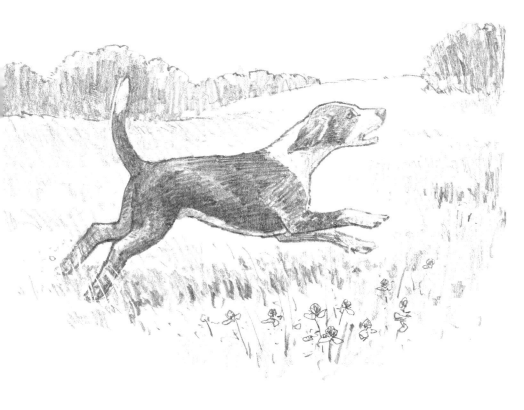

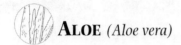

ALOE *(Aloe vera)*

Chemical Composition

A popular healing plant, aloe contains aloins, anthraquinones, and flavonoids.

Key Uses

The whole leaves and fresh or dehydrated juice from aloe are used mainly as a vulnerary (wound healer). This herb is an external demulcent and emollient (softening and soothing to the skin).

Current Research and Modern Uses

Internally, aloe is used when a strong cathartic (laxative with strong evacuant action) is indicated. Small doses act as an emmenagogue, increasing menstrual flow in human females.

Externally, the juice is used for burns, sunburn, wounds, insect bites, and so forth. It is one of the most effective healing agents for burns and injuries. Aloe relieves irritation as it heals.

Studies show that aloe has antibacterial and antifungal activity against a number of organisms, especially skin pathogens. It has proven activity against several viruses, including HIV-1. (Aloe reduces the amount of AZT required by as much as 90 percent.) Aloe has been approved, in injectable form, for veterinary use against fibrosarcomas and feline leukemia. The herb also enhances the function of the immune system and has anti-inflammatory and antiallergy activity.

Precautions and Side Effects

When aloe is taken internally, its laxative and cathartic effects can be dramatic. Since it stimulates uterine contractions, it should not be used internally during pregnancy. Aloe is also passed through the mother's milk, possibly exerting purgative effects on nursing animals.

Comments

I use aloe only externally; internal use has too much potential for adverse side effects. Aloe cannot be beaten as an external wound healer, especially for burns and superficial scrapes. I've found that some animals object to its application — possibly because of its astringent-like effects.

BLADDERWRACK *(Fucus vesiculosus)*

Chemical Composition

There are many species of seaweed or sea kelp (including hijiki, arame, kombu, and nori), and they are often used interchangeably with bladderwrack. Rich in algin, mannitol, carotene, and zeaxanthin, bladderwrack also contains polysaccharides, polyphenols, volatile oils, and other minerals, especially calcium.

Key Uses

The dried thallus or the whole plant is used as an antihypothyroid and a thyroid tonic. But it's also antirheumatic/antiarthritic, nutritive, and anti-inflammatory, and it stimulates metabolism.

Current Research and Modern Uses

Bladderwrack is used primarily for diseases of the thyroid, but it is also used to treat obesity, arteriosclerosis, and digestive disorders. For inflamed joints, it may be used both internally and externally (as a poultice). This seaweed provides building blocks needed by endocrine glands, making it helpful for endocrine imbalances. This is especially true in conditions affecting the female reproductive system.

Bladderwrack is an excellent food source and a wonderful supplement to the diet. It is rich in iodine. Recent work indicates that it may strengthen the immune system and, by this action, fight or prevent cancer.

Precautions and Side Effects

Allergic reactions have been known to occur with bladderwrack. Although the presence of too much iodine in the diet is said to possibly induce or worsen hyperthyroidism, you'd need to give your pet 33 pounds of seaweed daily to reach toxic levels.

Comments

In my practice, bladderwrack is a mainstay for hypothyroidism and many other glandular problems. I also think it's excellent for stimulating metabolism and reducing inflammation. Despite its fishy odor, not all animals enjoy the taste; camouflage it in food for a few days until your pet gets used to the flavor.

BURDOCK *(Arctium lappa)*

Chemical Composition

Burdock contains flavonoid glycosides, bitter glycosides, alkaloids, high amounts of inulin, vitamin
B_2, thiamin, iron, and silicon.

Key Uses

The roots, rhizomes, and seeds of burdock are used medicinally. The Chinese call the roots gobo. This herb is an alterative, diuretic,
and diaphoretic that is also nutritive. In addition, burdock is antioxidant
and antimicrobial.

Current Research and Modern Uses

Burdock root is a blood purifier; it's included in many formulas for toxin
elimination and bowel and lymphatic cleansing. It is often used to treat
arthritis and rheumatism. When taken as a tea or tincture, the root is
especially good for treating dry or scaly skin conditions, all forms of
eczema, and skin ailments related to arthritis.

Burdock promotes kidney function and cleans the liver. Recent studies
indicate that burdock has antibacterial and antifungal activity, possibly as
a function of its antioxidant biochemicals. One of its major constituents,
inulin, is anti-inflammatory and helps correct imbalances of the immune
system. Some evidence indicates antitumor activity in burdock, an action
that may be enhanced if burdock is combined with red clover.

Precautions and Side Effects

Rare cases of contact dermatitis from the leaves have been reported.
Internally, burdock has no known serious side effects, though diarrhea
may occur with extended use.

Comments

For its blood-cleansing capabilities and alterative powers, I add burdock
to most of my herbal prescriptions — especially for arthritis, skin problems of all kinds, and toxin-related conditions (particularly toxic or
chronic bowel syndrome). Use the chopped roots as a sprinkle or a tincture (for the finicky eater).

CALENDULA *(Calendula officinalis)*

Chemical Composition

The active constituents in calendula are saponins, carotenoids, bitter principles, essential oils, sterols, flavonoids, mucilage, and tocopherols. The fresh plant contains salicylic acid, which acts as an analgesic.

Key Uses

The flowers of calendula, which is often called pot marigold (not to be confused with the ornamental marigolds, *Tagetes* spp., that are commonly grown in flower gardens), help to stimulate wound healing. This herb is also a good astringent, liver-function enhancer, febrifuge (fever reducer), and tonic herb.

Current Research and Modern Uses

Many studies indicate that calendula flowers are antimicrobial, antifungal, antibacterial, antiviral, and vulnerary. They also stimulate the immune system, inhibit some tumors, have a calming effect on the nervous system, and aid liver function.

Externally, calendula is used for all types of wounds — cuts, scrapes, abrasions, burns, and inflammations of the mouth and pharynx. It is especially effective for wounds that heal poorly. Use it as a poultice on sprains and bruises.

Calendula promotes the reconstruction of tissue by enhancing fibroblastic growth; its anti-inflammatory activity decreases swelling and discharge as well as the scarring that normally occurs from burns, abscesses, and abrasions.

Precautions and Side Effects

Calendula is generally recognized to have no adverse side effects.

Comments

When made into a tea or ointment for use on open wounds, calendula is my favorite wound healer. It is so good, in fact, that I have to caution folks not to use it on wounds that need to drain (abscesses, for example), as they may heal over too quickly.

CATNIP *(Nepeta cataria)*

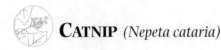

Chemical Composition

This herb is composed of essential oils, including cavracol, citronellol, neroli, geraniol, pulegone, thymol, nepetalactone, and nepetalic acid. It also has tannins, vitamins C and E, magnesium, manganese, and flavonoids.

Key Uses

In almost all animals, catnip acts as a sedative (in cats, the sedation is preceded by euphoric or aphrodisiac effects, a reaction not seen in dogs or other animals). It has nervine, carminative, antispasmodic, antipyretic, diaphoretic, and diuretic properties. The herb is also a stomachic (digestive tonic) and light emmenagogue, and it increases gallbladder activity.

Current Research and Modern Uses

The probable cause of a cat's blissful reaction to catnip is nepetalactone, a component of the essential oil that mimics a cat's sexual pheromones. Nepetalactone is also similar to the sedative constituents of valerian (see page 179), which may explain its sedative action in dogs and other animals.

Catnip has a mild tranquilizing effect on most animals, making it a good treatment for restlessness, nervousness, and insomnia. It is a gentle nervine that is also excellent for gastrointestinal upsets, such as colic, flatulence, diarrhea, and dyspepsia. Its diaphoretic activity makes it good for the early symptoms of colds, flus, and other feverish conditions, especially bronchitis.

Externally, catnip is used as an antiseptic poultice for sores and wounds. Dr. James Duke, a noted herbalist, has seen promising results using catnip to help prevent and slow the progression of cataracts.

Precautions and Side Effects

No significant side effects have been reported with catnip.

Comments

Catnip is a great calming herb. Most animals are susceptible to catnip's calming effects, but without the initial euphoria seen in cats. It has been my experience that most dogs respond better to valerian, St.-John's-wort, or chamomile than they do to catnip.

CAYENNE (*Capsicum* spp.)

Chemical Composition

The main constituents of cayenne are capsaicin; red coloring matter; and oleic, palmetic, and stearic acids. The herb is high in calcium, phosphorus, iron, and zinc as well as vitamins A, B, and C. (Its vitamin C content is greater per ounce than that of oranges, and it nearly doubles as the fruit ripens.)

Key Uses

Also known as chili pepper, the fresh and dried fruit of the cayenne plant is employed as a stimulant for all body systems. In addition, it has tonic, carminative, diaphoretic, rubefacient, hemostatic, and antioxidant properties.

Current Research and Modern Uses

Cayenne is an outstanding carrier herb that helps transport other herbs and medicines to various parts of the body, especially the heart, stomach, and brain. A useful systemic stimulant, cayenne regulates blood flow and strengthens the heart, arteries, capillaries, and nerves.

Cayenne is a general tonic that is also specific for the circulatory and digestive systems, and it balances blood pressure. In small amounts it aids digestion, stimulating the appetite and dispelling gas. It also eases the pains of arthritis and rheumatism and the itching of skin conditions. Cayenne can be used topically for those ailments as well.

In tests cayenne has been shown to slow the development of some cancers, possibly because of its high levels of vitamins and antioxidants.

Precautions and Side Effects

Very high doses of cayenne over long periods of time can cause problems, such as chronic gastritis, kidney and liver damage, and neurological effects. External applications may cause blistering.

Comments

Surprisingly, many pets have a hankering for spicy foods, making administration of cayenne easy. I find the herb especially helpful for treating arthritis pain, poor circulation, and heart conditions. I generally don't recommend topical applications, however.

CHAMOMILE (Roman, *Anthemus nobilis;* German, *Matricaria recutita*)

Chemical Composition

The volatile oil of chamomile contains chamazulene, isadol, mucilage, coumarin, and flavone glycosides.

Key Uses

Chamomile's flowers are an effective carminative, relieving gas and distention of the stomach. The plant is also anti-inflammatory, analgesic (pain relieving), and antiseptic. Its vulnerary action makes it an excellent topical wound healer.

Current Research and Modern Uses

Chamomile has a seemingly endless list of uses. Europeans have long used it to treat colic, diarrhea, insomnia, indigestion, toothache, swollen gums, skin problems, gout, sciatica, some cancers, and more. Perhaps the best indication of how Europeans feel about chamomile is the German saying *alles zutraut* — "capable of anything."

A gentle sedative that is safe for even young animals, chamomile can be used to alleviate anxiety, insomnia, and indigestion. Animal tests indicate that chamomile causes a reduction of aggressive behavior.

In addition to being effective against some bacteria and fungi, chamomile has anti-inflammatory activity that makes it ideal for inflamed eyes, sore throats, and other irritations. It is an excellent choice for gas, flatulence, and sore tummies, as well.

Precautions and Side Effects

No serious side effects or drug interactions are known. As with any herb, there is a small potential for sensitization.

Comments

Chamomile is my favorite sedative — one cup of tea, and I'm snoring in my favorite chair. It seems to work equally well with some pets. I like to add chamomile to topical treatments (in tea-spritzer, ointment, or oil-based forms) because I think it calms the irritable animal while healing the wound.

DANDELION *(Taraxacum officinale)*

Chemical Composition

Dandelion contains taraxacin (a crystalline bitter), taraxacerin (an acrid resin), and inulin. The roots and leaves contain variable amounts of vitamins A, C, E, and B complex; potassium (up to 5 percent); calcium; iron; thiamin; choline; lecithin; and riboflavin. The leaves have more beta-carotene than carrots do.

Key Uses

As a diuretic, dandelion stimulates the urinary organs. It's a tonic and general stimulant, especially for the urinary system and liver. The herb is also supportive of the liver and gallbladder, and it's used to treat gallstones.

Current Research and Modern Uses

In animal studies, dandelion has proved to be a strong diuretic, with an action comparable to that of the drug furosemide. But while furosemide depletes potassium from the body, dandelion resupplies it naturally.

Dandelion is one of the strongest cholagogues, increasing the liver's production of bile by more than 50 percent. In addition, the plant is a choleretic; it increases bile flow to the gallbladder. This benefits patients with colitis, liver congestion, gallstones, and several forms of liver insufficiency.

Precautions and Side Effects

There are virtually no reported side effects, but topical contact with the sap of the stems may produce allergic reactions in sensitive people. Since dandelion is a diuretic, remember to give your dog plenty of bathroom breaks during the day and evening.

Comments

In treating urinary disorders, I have had more luck using dandelion root than anything else. I add dandelion root to my herbal prescription for liver conditions or whenever I feel the whole body can use the stimulating action of this gentle tonic.

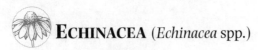

ECHINACEA (*Echinacea* spp.)

Chemical Composition

The *Echinacea* genus has an assortment of active constituents that can be divided into seven categories: polysaccharides, flavonoids, caffeic acid derivatives, essential oils, polyacetylenes, alkylamides, and miscellaneous chemicals. Amounts of the chemicals vary between leaf and root preparations, among different species, and at different times of the year.

Key Uses

Echinacea is the best choice to balance the immune system and is effective against all types of infections.

Current Research and Modern Uses

There is a vast amount of pharmacological information on echinacea. Studies have indicated that the herb elevates white blood cell count when it is low (but not when it is normal or high), promotes nonspecific T-lymphocyte activation, and enhances macrophage phagocytosis. It also has a mild, direct effect against bacteria, viruses, and yeasts. Most of the antimicrobial activity is probably due to its effects on the immune system.

Echinacea also promotes tissue regeneration and reduces inflammation. It possesses indirect anticancer activity via its general immuno-enhancing effects. In addition, echinacea has anti-inflammatory activity that helps alleviate rheumatoid arthritis.

Precautions and Side Effects

Echinacea is not toxic when used at recommended doses. In fact, chronic administration of the plant to rats at doses many times the human therapeutic dose produced no evidence of toxic effects. Mutagenic tests with echinacea demonstrated no cancer-causing activity.

Comments

I would not (and could not) practice holistic medicine without echinacea. In today's world I see mostly chronic diseases — arthritis, cancers, reactions to drugs — that I feel are immune-system related. Many of these conditions respond well to echinacea.

EYEBRIGHT (*Euphrasia officinalis*)

Chemical Composition

The main constituents of eyebright are glycosides (including aucubin), phenolic acid, tannins, resins, and volatile oil.

Key Uses

An astringent and anti-inflammatory, eyebright is also used as an anticatarrhal and expectorant.

Current Research and Modern Uses

Eyebright's best-known use is for conditions of the eye — particularly chronic inflammation, stinging and weeping eyes, and eyes that are overly sensitive to light. However, the herb can be used for treating infections of the mucous membranes, including sinusitis and nasal congestion.

Eyebright is effective when used internally as a tea or tincture, or externally as an eyewash.

Precautions and Side Effects

No serious adverse reactions have been reported.

Comments

Eyebright is simply the best medicine available for the red, irritated eye. I even use my animal eyewashes on myself! If I think an eye is infected, I usually add another antibiotic herb, such as elder, goldenrod, or goldenseal, to the mixture. For all eye infections, I like to use eyebright internally in combination with other antibiotic and toxin-cleansing herbs, such as echinacea, Oregon grape root, and possibly burdock root or cleavers.

GINGER *(Zingiber officinale)*

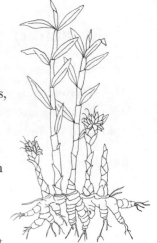

Chemical Composition

At least 477 chemicals — including essential oils, gingerols, shogaols, and phenolic compounds — have been isolated in ginger. Because the biochemicals are present in different concentrations in the fresh and dried plant, choose a combination of the two for the best effect.

Key Uses

The root of this Asian plant is used as a stimulant to revive and enhance the function of many organ systems. It's also an antispasmodic and carminative, and it can be applied topically as a rubefacient (to increase blood flow and heat in the treated region). As a diaphoretic, ginger increases circulation and sweating.

Current Research and Modern Uses

Ginger is an excellent herb for debilitated animals — particularly those with poor appetites; poor circulation and cold limbs; a deep, slow pulse; and general pallor. The herb's antispasmodic activity works to ease coughs, nausea, and pains of the stomach and lower back. It also helps alleviate all sorts of digestive problems, including diarrhea, colic, and flatulence.

Externally, ginger can be used as a poultice to treat muscle pains and strains and fibrositis. Ginger is mildly tonic to all organ systems.

Precautions and Side Effects

Because of its great warming ability, ginger should be used with caution in temperamental animals. The herb should be used in moderation during pregnancy.

Comments

Ginger is a wonder herb that's good for lots of ailments. But many animals don't like its taste, at least not initially. Animals that have been exposed to ginger's unique flavor during healthy periods appreciate it more on the days when they don't feel well.

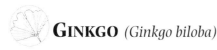

GINKGO *(Ginkgo biloba)*

Chemical Composition

This herb contains terpine lactones (or ginkgoglides) and flavone glycosides (flavonoids).

Key Uses

Ginkgo acts on two major systems of the body: the nervous and cardiovascular systems. Almost every medical condition that ginkgo successfully treats is due, at least in part, to poor circulation.

Current Research and Modern Uses

Dozens of human studies and hundreds of animal studies have confirmed ginkgo's medicinal effects. It enhances vitality by increasing blood flow to the brain, strengthening brain cells by acting as a free-radical scavenger, and making the transmission of nerve messages more effective. It is helpful in treating Alzheimer's disease, dementia (dimming mind syndrome), and depression. This herb enhances both long-term and short-term memory in youngsters and the elderly alike.

Ginkgo improves circulation by preventing or reducing the release of platelet-activating factor (PAF), the substance that increases stickiness. Ginkgo also helps maintain the integrity and elasticity of the blood vessels and reduces the tendency of vessels to contract and constrict (vasospasm) during times of stress.

Precautions and Side Effects

Ginkgo acts as a blood thinner; patients who are taking blood-thinning drugs (including aspirin) should not use ginkgo without first consulting a doctor or herbalist.

Rare side effects — including nausea, headache, dizziness, excessive bruising or bleeding from minor cuts, and bloodshot eyes — have been reported. (Interestingly, most patients note relief from headaches and dizziness while on ginkgo.) No particular adverse side effects have been found with long-term use. Patients often require several months of ginkgo use before results become noticeable.

GINSENG

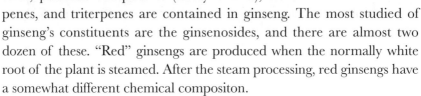

(Asian, *Panax ginseng;* American,
Panax quinquefolius; Siberian ginseng;
Eleutherococcus senticosus)

Chemical Composition

Saponins, sugars, lipids, vitamins, minerals, proteins, phenolic compounds (salicylic acid), ter-
penes, and triterpenes are contained in ginseng. The most studied of
ginseng's constituents are the ginsenosides, and there are almost two
dozen of these. "Red" ginsengs are produced when the normally white
root of the plant is steamed. After the steam processing, red ginsengs have
a somewhat different chemical compositon.

Key Uses

Ginseng is an adaptogenic and stimulant. This whole-body tonic is an
especially good cardiac stimulant.

Current Research and Modern Uses

Panax ginseng is considered the king of tonics — it supplies energy to the
entire body, helping it recover from stress, fatigue, weakness, and deficiencies. It is reported to have the power to move people to their physical
peak, increasing vitality as well as physical performance and mental
acuity. The ginsengs function as adaptogens; they restore normality and
increase nonspecific resistance to disease or other changes. Siberian ginseng was the original herb that was referred to as an adaptogen.

Comments

Ginseng is excellent for many ailments, but I do not prescribe it often for
several reasons. First, it's very difficult to know what you're getting when
you buy ginseng. Several studies have analyzed ginseng products from
Asia, and many of these products did not contain the amounts of the
herb stated on the label; some contained none. Second, there are several
species of ginseng, and each has a slightly different medicinal activity;
customers are often confused by the varieties. Third, our indigenous ginseng, *Panax quinquefolium,* is threatened by overharvesting in the wild.
Finally, ginseng is hard to grow, and it takes several years for the rootstock
to develop its full medicinal potential.

GOLDENSEAL *(Hydrastis canadensis)*

Chemical Composition

All parts of goldenseal, but especially the rhizome, contain several alkaloids: hydrastine, berberine, and canadine.

Key Uses

Goldenseal has many uses, mainly acting as an alterative, anti-inflammatory, astringent, antibiotic, antifungal, and cholagogue. It also has laxative, muscular stimulant, oxytocic (uterine stimulant), antitumor, and hemostatic properties.

Current Research and Modern Uses

Good for any inflammatory condition, goldenseal is especially helpful for inflammation of the mucous membranes (gastrointestinal, upper respiratory, urinary, reproductive, eye, mouth, throat, and sinus). This herb fights bacterial, viral, and fungal infections and can be used as an external wash for inflammation or infection of the eyes.

Use goldenseal for digestive problems and liver conditions. Goldenseal is valuable for treating loss of appetite, skin wounds or chronic skin conditions, infectious diarrhea, fevers, and lymph cleansing.

Precautions and Side Effects

Do not use goldenseal during pregnancy. The herb may alter blood pressure, and prolonged use (more than 2 weeks) alters the gut flora. High doses of goldenseal may interfere with vitamin-B metabolism, and the fresh plant can cause inflammation of mucous tissue in sensitive animals. In addition, some animals really dislike its taste.

Comments

Goldenseal is a wonder herb, but it is at risk of becoming an endangered species. If you can find a reliable source of organically grown goldenseal, by all means, use it. But if the label says "wildcrafted," please use Oregon grape root, an effective alternative.

HAWTHORN *(Crataegus laevigata)*

Chemical Composition

Hawthorn's major constituents are saponins, glycosides, flavonoids, acids (including ascorbic acid), and tannins. The berries also contain cardiotonic amines, choline and acetylcholine, and purine derivatives.

Key Uses

The ripe fruit of hawthorn is used as a cardiac tonic and hypotensive (to relax peripheral blood vessels). This herb is also astringent and diuretic.

Current Research and Modern Uses

Hawthorn is perhaps the world's best cardiotonic. It improves metabolic processes in the myocardium (which enhances the general function of the heart), dilates coronary blood vessels (thus improving coronary blood supply), and abolishes some types of rhythm disturbances. Hawthorn normalizes heart activity, either depressing or stimulating it, depending on the need. It is a good herb for heart failure or weakness.

Hawthorn is safer and milder in activity than digitalis, a popular medication. There are no cumulative effects with this herb (as with digitalis), and hawthorn may correct the undesirable side effects of that drug. The herb even has a synergistic effect with the medication; dosages of both can be reduced by about half when they are used in combination.

Hawthorn acts to stabilize collagen, resulting in decreased capillary permeability and fragility. In addition, the berries also strengthen appetite and digestion and are a good remedy for nervousness and insomnia.

Precautions and Side Effects

Health risks or adverse side effects from hawthorn have not been recorded. Since hawthorn potentiates the action of digitalis, consult an herbalist before taking hawthorn with it or any other cardiac drug.

Comments

If a patient has cardiac problems of any type, I recommend hawthorn. It is slow and gentle in its action, but it does not have adverse side effects.

KAVA KAVA *(Piper methysticum)*

Chemical Composition

The active ingredients of kava kava, found in the fat-soluble portion of the root and rhizome, include kava lactones or kava pyrones.

Key Uses

The rhizomes of kava kava, whose botanical name means "intoxicating pepper," are used to relieve anxiety and conditions related to tension and restlessness.

Current Research and Modern Uses

Kava kava, a plant native to the Pacific islands, relaxes the central nervous system without affecting mental sharpness; users actually exhibit improved memory and reaction time. Your pet won't build up a tolerance to the plant, so you won't need to keep increasing the dosage.

Studies have shown that kava kava creates changes in EEG patterns that are typical of antianxiety drugs — but without their sedative effects. It influences the brain's limbic system; researchers suspect that this action contributes to kava kava's muscle-relaxant and pain-reducing effects. The herb is a more potent analgesic than aspirin.

Kava kava can also be used to induce sleep. It is not a sedative but, rather, a hypnotic: It calms the mind and allows it to drift off, without any hangover the next morning. Used topically, kava kava acts as a local anesthetic, with effects comparable to those of the drug procaine. This plant is also effective against fungal skin infections.

Precautions and Side Effects

Kava kava can create mild gastrointestinal disturbances. Long-term or excessive use may cause a yellowing or rash of the skin or equilibrium problems. Consult an herbalist before using kava kava with barbiturates, antidepressants, or other drugs that act on the central nervous system. Do not use kava kava during pregnancy.

Comments

I use kava kava to help animals relax. I've found it especially helpful to calm nervous animals before athletic competitions or chiropractic adjustments.

LICORICE *(Glycyrrhiza glabra)*

Chemical Composition

The root of this plant contains glycosides (mainly glycyrrhizin), saponins, flavonoids, bitter principles, volatile oil, coumarins, asparagine, and estrogenic substances.

Key Uses

An adrenal-supporting herb, licorice is also used to soothe irritated membranes — especially those in the gastrointestinal tract (such as ulcers). This plant is an anti-inflammatory, antimicrobial, antiarthritic, tonic, and adaptogen (enhances the body's ability to adapt). It's often used to treat the liver and respiratory problems, such as bronchitis and coughs.

Current Research and Modern Uses

Glycyrrhizin, one of the plant's major active constituents, has a chemical structure similar to that of natural corticosteroids. Thus, licorice stimulates the secretion of hormones by the adrenal glands. The herb is an anti-inflammatory, reducing joint swelling and easing some skin conditions. Licorice raises the concentration of prostaglandins in the digestive system, promoting new cell growth and alleviating ulcers. It soothes irritated membranes and relieves abdominal colic by promoting mucus secretion in the stomach. It also prolongs stomach-cell life and decreases the secretion of pepsin.

Licorice root, which has antitussive, demulcent, and expectorant qualities, has long been used to alleviate coughs. It compares favorably to codeine in experiments. Research has also proved licorice root effective in treating liver toxicity. When the whole root (rather than an extract) is used, licorice acts as a tonic.

Precautions and Side Effects

Reported side effects include sodium retention and potassium loss, resulting in edema (accumulation of fluids within tissues); hypertension (high blood pressure); and hypokalemia (abnormally low potassium in the blood). Do not use licorice for patients with heart or liver disease or for patients who tend to retain sodium.

MILK THISTLE *(Silybum marianum)*

Chemical Composition

An important herb for liver ailments, milk thistle contains flavolignans (primarily silymarin, as well as silybin, silydianin, and silychristin), essential oils, bitter principles, and mucilage.

Key Uses

Milk thistle is the best available treatment for the liver. It also promotes milk secretion in the lactating female.

Current Research and Modern Uses

Few plant principles have been as extensively researched in recent years as milk thistle's primary active ingredient, silymarin. This chemical helps stabilize liver cell membranes and stimulates protein synthesis while also accelerating cell regeneration in liver tissue cells that are damaged by alcohol, drugs, and chronic liver disease.

Double-blind studies have shown milk thistle to be supportive in treating chronic inflammatory liver disorders, such as hepatitis, cirrhosis, and fatty infiltration of the liver. In addition, silymarin is considered a specific antidote for poisoning from the amanita (deathcap) mushroom. A few European studies even suggest that silymarin may help treat the scaly skin patches of psoriasis. Milk thistle is so safe that it can be used even by breast-feeding mothers.

Precautions and Side Effects

Rare mild laxative effects have been reported.

Comments

Milk thistle is without question the best therapy I have found for all sorts of liver conditions. Western medicine just does not have anything comparable. In addition to using it for specific liver maladies, I often add milk thistle to my herbal prescriptions because no matter what the disease, the liver is active in detoxification and metabolism.

MOTHERWORT *(Leonurus cardiaca)*

Chemical Composition

Motherwort is composed of bitter glycosides (including leonurin and leonuridine), alkaloids (including leonuinine and stachydrene), volatile oil, and tannins.

Key Uses

Motherwort's aerial parts, which are gathered at flowering, have cardiac tonic properties. The herb is also known for promoting menstruation and acting as a sedative and antispasmodic.

Current Research and Modern Uses

Motherwort is primarily used as as a support for the female reproductive system and as a cardiac tonic to strengthen the heart without straining it. While motherwort is a specific herb for an overrapid heart rate, it is also good for most heart conditions, especially those associated with anxiety and tension. Motherwort is much like valerian — it is hypotensive and sedative.

Motherwort is not really a uterine tonic; rather, it works more as a uterine stimulant. This herb is used during the first stages of pregnancy to prepare the uterus for childbirth and in the later stages of pregnancy to ease childbirth and promote contractions. It is also a useful tonic for menopausal changes.

Precautions and Side Effects

No serious side effects have been reported. Sensitive patients may develop contact dermatitis from exposure to the leaves or flowers.

Comments

For heart problems I think of hawthorn first; then I consider motherwort. I think some patients can use its added sedative effects. I recommend motherwort for some of my spayed female patients with heart conditions, because spaying creates a condition similar to that which occurs in human women at menopause.

I do occasionally take motherwort myself, hoping for a part, if not all, of the 300-year life span enjoyed by a Chinese sage who drank motherwort tea every day.

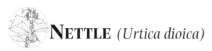

NETTLE *(Urtica dioica)*

Chemical Composition

Nettle contains indoles, including histamine and serotonin; formic acid; chlorophyll; glucoquinine; iron; vitamins A, C, and K; acetylcholine; silicon; protein; and fiber.

Key Uses

Also known as stinging nettle, the leaves of this herb are nutritive, supplying important vitamins and minerals to the whole body. Its tonic effects are well known among herbalists. Nettle is also a diuretic, galactagogue (enhancing milk production), hemostatic, and astringent.

Current Research and Modern Uses

As a general tonic, nettle strengthens, supports, and provides nutrients to the whole body. Because of its high iron content, it is beneficial for treating anemia.

The root offers good antibiotic possibilities; its high sterol levels enhance the production of white blood cells. A poultice of the astringent leaves may be used for nosebleeds or other hemorrhagic conditions, such as uterine bleeding.

This herb has been used for a variety of urinary complaints, including urinary stones, nephritis, cystitis, and the swelling of benign prostatic hyperplasia (BPH). Other conditions that have been successfully treated with nettle include eczema and other skin conditions, arthritis, rheumatism, stomach problems, and lung ailments, such as asthma.

Precautions and Side Effects

No serious side effects are known, but a few rare allergic reactions have been observed. Unless handled carefully with gloved hands, the fresh leaves — which have sharp, barblike projections — can cause a stinging sensation. Cooked and dried leaves lose this property.

Comments

One of my favorite nutritive herbs, nettle is a great general tonic. It makes a tasty tea and sprinkle that most animals take when it is added to their food.

OAT *(Avena sativa)*

Chemical Composition

The active ingredients of oat are soluble oligosac-
charides and polysaccharides, salicylic acid,
steroid saponins, amino acids, magnesium, calcium,
and flavonoids.

Key Uses

The fresh or dried aboveground parts of oats are most frequently employed, but other parts are also used: the milky,
still-green fruits; the ripe, dried fruits; and the dried leaf and
stem. Oat makes an excellent nervine tonic, and it even has
antidepressant properties. Oat is also nutritive, demulcent, and
vulnerary.

Current Research and Modern Uses

Oat is one of the best remedies for feeding the nervous system (either
alone or in combination with other nervines), especially when it is under
stress. The herb is used as a tonic to balance the mind, body, and spirit.
Oat is considered a specific in cases of nervous debility and exhaustion
associated with depression, as well as for general debility. Recently, this
herb has been used as a sexual tonic for both males and females.

Externally, oat makes a wonderfully soothing remedy for skin conditions. Several oat bath products for animals are commercially available,
but you can easily make your own. Boil about 1 pound of shredded,
organic oat straw in 2 quarts of water for about ½ hour. Strain the liquid
and add it to your pet's bathwater, just before the final rinse.

Precautions and Side Effects

No health problems have been associated with oat.

Comments

I add oat to almost all my herbal prescriptions because most sick animals
are anxious about their conditions. The herb is also readily accepted by
most animals, especially in the form of oatmeal.

OREGON GRAPE (*Mahonia* spp.)

Chemical Composition

A good source of berberine and several other alkaloids (including hydrastine), Oregon grape also
contains resins and tannins.

Key Uses

This plant has strong antibiotic and skin-healing effects. It
stimulates bile production, has immune-stimulating activity,
and lowers fevers. *Note:* At the present time, most herbalists substitute
Oregon grape root for goldenseal, which is being wild-harvested to the
point of near extinction. The two herbs have similar components, and
Oregon grape root may actually be better for skin conditions.

Current Research and Modern Uses

Oregon grape root is used to treat infections and inflammations that
affect the mucous membranes of the respiratory, digestive, and genitouri-
nary tracts. Berberine, a major constituent of the plant, has broad-spec-
trum activity against bacteria, protozoans, fungi, and yeasts. It also
inhibits adherence of Group A streptococcal bacteria to host cells.

Oregon grape root stimulates the immune system by activating
macrophages and increasing blood supply to the spleen. In human and
rat studies, Oregon grape root demonstrated an activity against brain
tumors (by stimulating white blood cells) that is stronger than that of the
currently used chemotherapy agents.

Precautions and Side Effects

Oregon grape root is generally nontoxic at recommended dosages. Do
not use it during pregnancy, however. High doses may interfere with the
metabolism of B vitamins.

Comments

Oregon grape root might not be quite as strong as antibiotic drugs, but
since berberine is effective against yeast, I see none of the bothersome
yeast overgrowths that occur with antibiotic use. For prolonged periods, I
recommend the addition of natural "good-guy" bugs, such as lactobacilli,
supplied in yogurt or in supplement form.

RED CLOVER *(Trifolium pratense)*

Chemical Composition

Red clover contains phenolic glycosides, flavonoids, coumarin derivatives, cyanogenic glycosides, vitamins and minerals, and volatile oils (methyl salicylate and others). The herb also has isoflavones, which possess estrogen-like activity.

Key Uses

The blossoms of red clover are used as an alterative, expectorant, and antispasmodic. They also promote skin healing and may have antitumor activity.

Current Research and Modern Uses

As an alterative, red clover is used to treat a wide range of skin conditions, such as eczema, eruptions, and psoriasis. An expectorant, red clover is helpful for treating coughs and bronchitis. It has a mild, relaxing nervine quality and can be used along with or in place of chamomile.

Red clover is what herbalists refer to as a blood purifier, which means it helps remove accumulated toxins. Research suggests that the herb may have anticancer effects in animals, perhaps because of its high levels of carotene and vitamin E. Most herbalists, when treating cancers of various types, combine red clover with other suitable herbs.

Precautions and Side Effects

No side effects are known when the herb is used at recommended doses. Because of its high coumarin levels (coumarin inhibits blood clotting) and estrogenic-like compounds, I am cautious when using red clover in pregnant patients or those with bleeding disorders.

Comments

Red clover is another one of those herbs that is "good for what ails you," and it's readily accepted by most animals either as a tea or food sprinkle. I almost always combine red clover with burdock root because the two seem to act synergistically. All my cancer patients take red clover in combination with other appropriate herbs.

SARSAPARILLA (*Smilax* spp.)

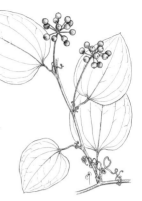

Chemical Composition

Sarsaparilla is recognized for its steroid saponins, including sarsaponin, smilasaponin, and sarsaparilloside; and its aglycones, including sarsasapogenin, smilagenin, and pollinastanol. The herb also contains starch, resins, and a trace of volatile oil.

Key Uses

The roots and rhizomes of sarsaparilla are anti-inflammatory, making the herb particularly good for skin diseases. It also has antiarthritic properties, which may stem from the anti-inflammatory effects. As a diaphoretic and antipyretic, sarsaparilla causes sweating and lowers fevers. It's also a diuretic, alterative, and tonic, enhancing the balance of all body systems.

Current Research and Modern Uses

Sarsaparilla is used most often for chronic diseases, such as arthritis and skin conditions. It is especially good for scaly skin conditions, including psoriasis and eczema, in which there is a lot of irritation.

The saponins in sarsaparilla bind bacterial toxins in the gut — this is possibly due to its activity as a blood purifier, alterative, and antipyretic. The herb has been used as a male reproductive-system stimulant, but this use is questionable. While it contains chemicals that can be converted to testosterone in a test tube, it's doubtful that conversion can occur in the body.

Precautions and Side Effects

No serious side effects are known to have occurred with the use of sarsaparilla, but stomach upset and kidney irritation may occur in rare cases.

Comments

I try to include sarsaparilla, which is readily accepted by most animals, in all herbal prescriptions for skin ailments and chronic arthritic conditions. Because it is an alterative and blood cleanser, it's good in combination with such herbs as burdock and yellow dock.

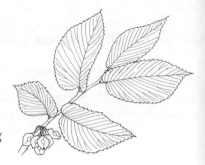

SLIPPERY ELM *(Ulmus rubra)*

Chemical Composition

With mucilage similar to that in mucilage-rich linseed, slippery elm coats, soothes, protects, and rejuvenates areas suffering from infection, inflammation, and other irritants.

Key Uses

Slippery elm soothes irritated mucous membranes and eases diarrhea. It's also used internally for stomach ulcers, colitis, sore throats, and coughs and topically for wounds and abscesses.

Current Research and Modern Uses

Native Americans used slippery elm bark for dysentery, diarrhea, and ulcers. They also used a topical poultice of the herb to treat sores and wounds. The USDA currently lists slippery elm bark as a safe and effective demulcent (a substance that provides a protective coating and soothes irritated tissues) that can be taken orally.

Precautions and Side Effects

Prolonged use (more than 3 weeks) in high dosages may overcoat the intestinal tract and prevent absorption of nutrients.

Comments

Slippery elm is absolutely the best remedy I've come across for the animal with a nervous stomach. No one traveling with a pet should be without it. The show animal who frets before a performance will almost certainly benefit from a dose of slippery elm. I also use this herb in combination with other modalities, such as homeopathy and acupuncture, when treating more severe cases of intestinal upset — colitis, ulcerative colitis, ulcers, and so on.

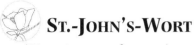

ST.-JOHN'S-WORT

(Hypericum perforatum)

Chemical Composition

St.-John's-wort contains numerous compounds with documented biological activity, the naphthodi-anthrones hypericin and pseudohypericin, a broad range of flavonoids, essential oils, and xanthones.

Key Uses

This popular antidepressant is also an antiviral. When used topically and in oral tinctures, St.-John's-wort has wound-healing capabilities.

Current Research and Modern Uses

St.-John's-wort is one of the most scientifically studied and most used herbs (especially in Germany) in today's herbal pharmacopeia. At least two dozen randomized trials conducted on several thousand humans with mild to moderately severe depressive disorders have shown responses to St.-John's-wort that are as good as or better than those seen with currently available pharmaceutical antidepressives.

Two of the plant's constituents, hypericin and pseudohypericin, inhibit a variety of encapsulated viruses, including herpes simplex type 1 and 2, human HIV-1, murine cytomegalovirus, and parainfluenza-3 virus. In addition, hypericin prevents tumor cell growth and induces tumor cell death by inhibiting protein kinase C. An excellent wound healer, hypericin extracts appear to have an antibacterial action against gram-positive organisms and also increase new cell formation.

Precautions and Side Effects

St.-John's-wort extract seems to be relatively free of side effects. The most frequently noted side effects are gastrointestinal irritation, allergic reaction, fatigue, and restlessness. St.-John's-wort is known to cause photosensitization (and occasionally loss of appetite, nervousness, coma, and possibly death) in cattle, horses, rabbits, sheep, and swine. I have not found reports of photosensitization in dogs, but I always advise clients who have light-skinned dogs to keep them out of bright sunlight while their pets are using St.-John's-wort.

TURMERIC *(Curcuma longa)*

Chemical Composition

Turmeric is a member of the ginger family, and it contains a mix of phenolics called curcumin. Other active ingredients include volatile oil (with tumerone and zingiberene), cineole and other monoterpenes, sugars, starch, protein, and high amounts of vitamin A and other vitamins and minerals.

Key Uses

The rhizome of turmeric is used as an antioxidant and anti-inflammatory. It's a good choice for liver conditions, irritable bowel syndrome, and other gastrointestinal problems. Turmeric is an antimicrobial and anti-carcinogen that is used for cardiovascular ailments.

Current Research and Modern Uses

Turmeric has liver-protecting properties: It stimulates the flow of bile (increasing output by as much as 100 percent) and increases its solubility.

Tests indicate that the anti-inflammatory effects of turmeric are comparable to those of cortisone and phenylbutazone. In addition, turmeric has long been used as a carminative for decreasing gas formation; reducing intestinal spasms; and increasing secretion of secretin, gastrin, bicarbonate, and pancreatic enzymes.

The positive cardiovascular effects of turmeric include lowered cholesterol levels, inhibited platelet aggregation, interference with intestinal cholesterol uptake, increased conversion of cholesterol into bile acids, and increased excretion of bile acids.

Turmeric has potential as an anticancer herb. It interferes in all steps of cancer formation: initiation, promotion, and progression.

Precautions and Side Effects

No toxicity has been reported at normal intake levels. With very high amounts, inflammation or ulceration of the stomach lining may occur.

Comments

While most culinary herbs have medicinal value, turmeric has potent therapeutic activities against a wide variety of ailments. It's also easy to dose for most pets; simply sprinkle some over their food.

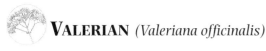

VALERIAN *(Valeriana officinalis)*

Chemical Composition

Another famous herb, valerian contains volatile oils (valepotriates, valerianic acid, valeranone, and valernal), esters, and alkaloids.

Key Uses

Valerian is used as a nervine tonic to calm nervous disorders from tension, anxiety, and discomfort. It's an antispasmodic, sedative, and pain reliever that is also good for upset stomachs.

Current Research and Modern Uses

Recent studies have shown that this herb sedates and regulates the autonomic nervous system and relieves tension and restlessness. When used in animals, valerian typically decreases unrest, anxiety, and aggressiveness without decreasing reaction time. Oddly, reaction time is actually improved with valerian.

A primary sedative for sleep disorders associated with anxiety, nervousness, exhaustion, headache, and hysteria, valerian acts as a tranquilizer that calms nervous-system imbalances, both physical and psychological. Many studies confirm the herb's usefulness for insomnia, but not all cases of insomnia respond to valerian. The herb is rapidly metabolized; the effects are gone by morning, leaving no side effects or morning "hangover."

Precautions and Side Effects

The whole root (rather than an extract) of valerian is virtually without toxicity. Approximately 5 percent of people respond to valerian with hyperactivity. If this occurs in your pet, simply discontinue use.

Comments

I find valerian very effective for most animals with separation anxiety or insomnia — the nighttime pacer, whiner, and crier. I like to use it both before and after surgery or during any prolonged disease, the times when Pet is the most anxious.

YARROW *(Achillea millefolium)*

Chemical Composition

Yarrow's active ingredients include volatile oils, sesquiterpene lactones, alkamids, flavones, and a bitter substance called achilleine.

Key Uses

The flowers and leaves of yarrow are used to stop blood flow. The plant is also used for loss of appetite; for liver, gall-bladder, and stomach complaints; and as an antipyretic. In addition, yarrow is antiseptic, anti-inflammatory, analgesic, and diaphoretic. The flowers are thought to have more potent medicinal qualities than the leaves.

Current Research and Modern Uses

The common name soldier's wound wort is a key to yarrow's primary external use — to stop the bleeding and infection of "battle wounds," such as cuts, scrapes, and abrasions. A poultice of the flowers and leaves stems blood flow from a fresh wound, as long as it is not bleeding profusely.

Internally, yarrow is used to aid the liver, soothe upset stomachs, and improve poor digestion. It is probably one of the best herbs for lowering fevers. Traditionally, yarrow has also been used to treat inflammatory conditions of the joints.

Precautions and Side Effects

Yarrow may cause contact dermatitis. It can also cause photosensitization and other allergic reactions.

Comments

I've mostly used yarrow as an external wound dressing. In my part of the country, yarrow grows wild in most of the pasturelands that are riddled with rocks and flint outcroppings. Thus, the herb is readily available when we (and our rambunctious grandkids) fall and are most likely to need it.

Some of my holistic veterinary friends have used yarrow internally more than I have, and many of them have found it to be an excellent herb for fevers, colds, and flulike symptoms.

YELLOW DOCK *(Rumex crispus)*

Chemical Composition

Yellow dock's primary chemical constituents are anthro-quinone glycosides, tannins, and oxalic acid. It is also high in iron, vitamins, and thiamine.

Key Uses

Used to treat dry, itchy skin, yellow dock is also a blood cleanser.

Current Research and Modern Uses

Yellow dock is typically used as an alterative (blood cleanser), but investigations into this use haven't uncovered any one cause for its successful clinical applications. The herb's thiamine content is one suspected reason. Yellow dock also has mild antibacterial activities.

Of all the herbs, yellow dock has one of the strongest reputations for clearing up skin problems, liver and gallbladder ailments (Native Americans used it to treat jaundice), and glandular inflammation and swelling. Its high iron content makes it an effective treatment for anemia. Conditions that respond well to yellow dock include eczema, ringworm, psoriasis, and cancer.

Precautions and Side Effects

No side effects have been reported at recommended doses. The oxalic acid in yellow dock's leaves and roots, if taken in large doses, may be irritating to the intestinal tract.

Comments

In my practice I recommend yellow dock — often in combination with other herbs, such as licorice root and Oregon grape root — for all skin-related problems. I also use yellow dock whenever I think blood cleansing would benefit the patient. Most of my patients with chronic conditions benefit from a general detox formula that includes yellow dock.

Other Useful Herbs

ARTICHOKE *(Cynara scolymus)*

The fresh or dried leaves of artichoke are used as a liver tonic and protective, with damage-preventing properties similar to those of milk thistle. This popular food stimulates the regeneration of liver cells and is also a bitter. It protects the body from toxins, restores healthy growth of liver cells, increases the amount of bile available for digestion, and reduces blood cholesterol and other fats. And it's generally recognized as safe with no known toxicity. If your pet doesn't like the taste of milk thistle or turmeric, artichoke is a good alternative.

BLACK COHOSH *(Cimicifuga racemosa)*

The dried roots and rhizomes of black cohosh contain resin, bitter glycosides, ranunculin, salicylic acid, tannin, and phytoestrogens. Black cohosh's primary use is as a normalizer and relaxant for the female reproductive tract. It may also be used for arthritic and rheumatic pains and to reduce spasms associated with coughs. For reproductive problems it combines well with blue cohosh. No health hazards are known to exist with proper use.

Most often I use black cohosh in combination with other reproductive herbs — dong quai, blue cohosh, wild yam, vitex, motherwort, and secondary herbs — as well as acupuncture and other alternative methods. I have been pleased with black cohosh's results for a variety of female problems.

BUGLEWEED *(Lycopus virginicus, L. europaeus)*

The aerial parts of bugleweed are specific for the overactive thyroid; they inhibit the peripheral deoidination of the thyroid hormone thyroxin. This herb will also aid a weak heart when there is an associated buildup of water in the body, and it acts as a sedative for cough relief, especially when the cough is of a nervous nature.

DONG QUAI *(Angelica sinensis)*

Dong quai is also known as Chinese angelica; the roots and rhizomes of this plant are used as a uterine tonic, antispasmodic, and alterative. Sometimes called the "female ginseng," dong quai is used in human medicine to treat almost all female gynecological ailments, especially menstrual cramps, irregularity, it delayed flow, and weakness. It is also a good herb to relieve the symptoms of menopause. In general, dong quai is an excellent tonic for the reproductive tract. In addition, it is an antispas-modic for insomnia, hypertension, and cramps. It is nourishing to the blood, making it a useful blood purifier and treatment for anemia.

Dong quai can cause photosensitivity. Do not use the herb during pregnancy or for patients with diabetes.

IRISH MOSS *(Chondrus crispus)*

Like bladderwrack, Irish moss is a seaweed. The dried thallus contains carrageenins, iodine, bromine, iron, other mineral salts, vitamins A and B_1, and up to 80 percent mucilage. This herb is an expectorant and demulcent used mainly for respiratory problems such as bronchitis. It is also used for digestive conditions such as gastritis and ulcers, and it has been applied topically to sores and ulcers. The carrageenin in Irish moss is used as a binding agent in the food industry to make jellies, aspic, and other products, and in the cosmetics industry as a skin softener.

Irish moss is commonly prepared as syrup in combination with Iceland moss *(Cetraria islandica)* and blackstrap molasses.

MULLEIN *(Verbascum thapsus)*

The leaves, flowers, and occasionally roots of the roots are used as a demulcent, anodyne, antispasmodic, astringent, mild diuretic, expectorant, nonnarcotic analgesic, mild sedative, and vulnerary. This plant is most useful for treating ailments of the lungs, such as coughs, sore throat, and bronchitis; ears, particularly infections; urinary tract, including infections and incontinence; stomach, especially cramps and intestinal catarrh; and nervous system, to induce sleep and relieve pain and headaches. Although the fine hairs on the leaves and flowers of mullein can be irritating to some, this problem is eliminated by straining the tea or tincture before use.

PARSLEY *(Petroselinum crispum)*

Parsley is a breath freshener, diuretic, and mild laxative that has hypoten-sive and antimicrobial properties. It has also been used to treat liver prob-lems and gallstones. Its estrogenic qualities help promote menstruation and milk production. Parsley is a good herb to use after meals to prevent bad breath. However, make sure that Pet does not have any underlying conditions, such as dental problems or digestive upsets, that may be caus-ing halitosis.

Do not use parsley during pregnancy. The herb may cause nerve inflammation if used to excess.

SAW PALMETTO *(Serenoa repens)*

This herb's primary effects are on the digestive tract, stimulating the appetite and increasing body weight. It also has calming qualities that are good for Pet's general health and disposition. Saw palmetto is frequently used to tone and strengthen the male reproductive system and as a treatment for benign prostatic hyperplasia (BHP) and infections of the prostate and urogenital organs.

No side effects have been reported when saw palmetto is used as recommended. Stomach complaints, though rare, may occur.

THYME *(Thymus* spp.)

Thyme has expectorant, antispasmodic, antimicrobial, astringent, and carminative qualities. It is a good remedy for coughs, asthma, and chronic or acute bronchitis, and also treats dyspepsia and sluggish digestion. When used externally, its strong antiseptic properties help heal wounds.

Because thyme is a uterine stimulant, it should not be used during pregnancy. Skin sensitivity is also a possibility when it is used externally.

WALNUT *(Juglans* spp.)

Walnut has astringent and anthelmintic properties. In Europe, the herb is a popular remedy for skin and eye conditions. I use walnut flower essence quite often for animals undergoing transitions, such as a move to a new home, the loss of a companion, the addition of a new member to the family, or any form of physical or emotional change.

The herb may cause digestive disorders with prolonged use.

YUCCA *(Yucca* spp.)

Although yucca is used to treat liver and gallbladder disorders, arthritis, hip dyspasia, and joint injuries, research substantiating its efficacy has not been conclusive. I occasionally employ yucca for short-term use in cases of arthritis. However, I have not been impressed with the consistency of the results. While I have never seen any problems with yucca, I am cautious to watch for intestinal complaints.

Yucca can be purgative and cause intestinal cramping. Long-term use may slow the absorption of fat-soluble vitamins.

Glossary

Adaptogen. A nontoxic agent that increases an organism's ability to adapt. Adaptogenic herbs work well with other herbs (and other medicines), generally adding to their activities.

Alterative. Acts as a blood purifier, gradually restoring the body to its proper state of health and vitality. Alteratives are used to treat toxicity of the blood, infections, arthritis, cancer, and skin eruptions. Alteratives also help the body assimilate nutrients and eliminate the waste products of metabolism.

Analgesic. Able to reduce pain.

Anthelmintic. Able to destroy or expel worms from the digestive tract.

Antiabortive. Helps inhibit the termination of a pregnancy.

Antiasthmatic. Relieves symptoms of asthma by dilating bronchioles or breaking up mucus.

Antibiotic. Inhibits the growth of or destroys microorganisms, including bacteria, viruses, protozoans, and fungi. While herbal antibiotics often have direct germ-killing effects, many of them also stimulate the body's own immune response.

Anticatarrhal. Helps the body remove excess mucus buildup, whether in the sinuses or in other parts of the body.

Antiemetic. Reduces nausea to relieve or prevent vomiting.

Antifungal. Inhibits fungal infestations.

Anti-inflammatory. Inhibits inflammation.

Antilithic. *See* **Lithotriptics.**

Antipyretic. Reduces or prevents fevers.

Antirheumatic. An agent used for the symptomatic treatment of rheumatism.

Antiseptic. An agent applied to the skin to prevent the growth of microorganisms.

Antispasmodic. Prevents or relaxes muscle spasms or cramps.

Antitussive. Prevents or inhibits coughs.

Antiviral. Inhibits viral infections.

Aphrodisiac. Increases sexual potency, appetite, or sensitivity.

Aromatic. Having a strong and often pleasant odor that can stimulate the digestive system. Aromatics are often used to add aroma and taste to other medicinals.

Astringent. An agent with a constricting or binding effect. Astringents are commonly used to stop hemorrhages, discharges, and secretions and to treat swollen tissues.

Bitter. A bitter-tasting herb that acts as a stimulant for the digestive system through the taste buds.

Cardiotonic. Increases heart tone and function.

Carminative. Relieves intestinal gas and severe pains of the bowels. Carminatives are rich in volatile oils, which stimulate peristalsis of the digestive system and relax the stomach.

Cathartic or laxative. Clears the bowels.

Cholagogue. Promotes the flow of bile into the small intestine. Cholagogues also have a laxative effect, since bile is our internally produced, all-natural laxative.

Demulcent. Soothes irritated membranes, especially mucous membranes.

Diaphoretic. Induces sweating, thus aiding the skin in the elimination of toxins.

Diuretic. Increases the secretion and elimination of urine. Diuretics help eliminate internal toxins and treat water retention, lymph swellings, infections of the urinary tract, skin conditions, and stones and gravel of the urinary system.

Emetic. Induces vomiting and causes the stomach to empty.

Emmenagogue. Promotes or regulates menstruation, stimulating and normalizing menstrual flow. Emmenagogues also act as tonics to the female reproductive system.

Emollients. When applied to the skin, emollients soften, soothe, or protect.

Expectorant. Expels mucus from the lungs and throat.

Febrifuge. *See* **Antipyretic.**

Galactogogue. Increases the flow of milk in a nursing female.

Hemostatic. Arrests hemorrhaging.

Hepatic. Tones and strengthens the liver and increases the flow of bile. *See also* **Cholagogue.**

Hypnotic. Induces sleep without inducing a hypnotic trance.

Laxative. *See* **Cathartic.**

Lithotriptic. Helps dissolve and eliminate urinary and biliary stones and gravel.

Mucilage. Gelatinous constituents of herbs that act as demulcents and emollients.

Nervine. Tones and strengthens the nervous system. Some nervines act as stimulants; some act as relaxants.

Oxytocic. Stimulates contraction of the uterus.

Parasiticide. *See* **Anthelmintic.**

Pectoral. Strengthens and heals the respiratory system.

Purgative. *See* **Cathartic.**

Rubefacient. When applied to the skin, rubifacients cause a gentle local irritation and stimulation and dilation of the capillaries, thus increasing circulation to the region. Rubifacients draw inflammation and congestion from deeper areas, making them useful for the treatment of sprains, arthritis, rheumatism, and other problems involving the joints.

Sedative. Calms the nervous system and reduces stress and nervousness throughout the body.

Sialagogue. Stimulates the flow of saliva, aiding in the digestion of starches.

Soporific. Sleep-producing herbs. *See also* **Hypnotics.**

Stimulant. Increases the activity of a specific organ system or the whole body.

Styptic. Stops external bleeding through astringency. *See also* **Astringent.**

Tonic. Strengthens and enlivens specific organs or the whole body. Most tonics have general effects on the whole body, but they also typically have a marked effect on a specific organ system.

Vulnerary. When applied externally, vulneraries aid in the healing of wounds and cuts by promoting cell growth and repair.

Organ System Tonic Herbs

ORGAN SYSTEM	TONIC HERBS
Immune system	Astragalus, echinacea, ginseng (all species), licorice, schisandra
Nervous system	Chamomile, ginkgo, Siberian ginseng, hop, lemon balm, lobelia, passionflower, peppermint, skullcap, valerian
Cardiovascular system	Bugleweed, cayenne, Siberian ginseng, hawthorn, kelp, motherwort, rosemary, turmeric, valerian
Musculoskeletal system	Alfalfa, devil's claw, echinacea, horsetail, licorice, sarsaparilla, saw palmetto, wild yam, yarrow
Liver and biliary	Dandelion, goldenseal, Oregon grape, parsley, rhubarb, sassafras, wild yam
Digestive system	Artichoke, dandelion, gentian, ginger, milk thistle, turmeric
Female reproductive system	Black cohosh, black haw, cramp bark, chaste tree, dong quai, ginger, licorice, red raspberry, valerian
Male reproductive system	Burdock, damiana, Siberian ginseng, licorice, pumpkin seed, pygeum, sarsaparilla, saw palmetto

Herbs for Specific Conditions

Before you begin using a remedy listed here, be sure that you read all about the herb in part 3. Also, consult the chapters on specific conditions for more information.

CONDITION	INTERNAL HERBS	EXTERNAL HERBS
Abscess	Cayenne, cleavers, echinacea, garlic, goldenseal, marsh mallow root, oregano	Calendula, chamomile, comfrey, lavender, marsh mallow root, plantain, St-John's-wort, yarrow
Acne	Burdock root, cleavers, dandelion root, echinacea, licorice root, red clover, sarsaparilla	
Allergic rhinitis (see Upper respiratory disease)		
Allergies	Astragalus, dandelion root, echinacea, fenugreek, goldenseal, licorice root, milk thistle, nettle, Oregon grape root, thyme, turmeric	
Anxiety	Catnip, chamomile, hop, kava kava, lavender, oat, passionflower, St.-John's-wort, skullcap, valerian	
Arrhythmia (see Cardiovascular disease)		
Arthritis	Antiarthritics: alfalfa, devil's claw, frankincense, turmeric, yucca; For pain and inflammation: cayenne, feverfew, licorice root, St.-John's-wort, willow bark, wild yam; Antioxidants: basil, celery seed, ginger, oregano, parsley, thyme	
Asthma	Astragalus, ginkgo, licorice, mullein	
Bacterial or viral infection	Calendula, cat's claw, chaparral, echinacea, elder, garlic, ginger, goldenseal, lavender, licorice root, myrrh, oregano, Oregon grape root, Pau d'arco, rose, rosemary, St.-John's-wort, thyme, yarrow	
Bad breath	Dill, fennel, parsley	

CONDITION	INTERNAL HERBS	EXTERNAL HERBS
Bladder infection (see Urinary tract infection)		
Bladder stones (see Urinary tract infection)		
Blepharitis (see Conjunctivitis)		
Bronchitis	Astragalus, coltsfoot, echinacea, goldenseal, licorice root, marsh mallow, mullein, Oregon grape root, osha root, plantain, thyme	
Burns		Aloe (for pain, add a pinch of echinacea and/or kava kava) or make a poultice of one or more of the following: calendula, chamomile, comfrey, plantain, St.-John's-wort)
Cardiovascular disease	Heart specifics: hawthorn, motherwort; Diuretics: dandelion root; Heart supporters: cayenne, ginger, ginkgo, *Panax ginseng;* Nervines: oat	
Cataracts	Bilberry, eyebright; Antioxidants: basil, celery seed, ginger, oregano, parsley, thyme	Eyebright
Circulatory problems	Cayenne, ginger, ginkgo	
Cognitive dysfunction (dimming mind syndrome)	Ginkgo, Siberian ginseng	
Colic	Aniseed, caraway, cardamom, catnip, cayenne, chamomile, cinnamon, coriander, dill, fennel, ginger, licorice root, peppermint, valerian	
Colitis	Chamomile, licorice root, marsh mallow, peppermint, slippery elm	
Conjunctivitis	Bilberry, echinacea, eyebright, goldenseal, Oregon grape root	Calendula, chamomile, eyebright
Constipation	Aloe, cascara sagrada, flaxseed, licorice root, senna, slippery elm, yellow dock	

CONDITION	INTERNAL HERBS	EXTERNAL HERBS
Cough	Coltsfoot, licorice root, mullein, osha root, plantain, red sage, thyme	
Cuts and scrapes		Aloe, calendula, chamomile, chickweed, cleavers, comfrey, elder, garlic, goldenseal, lavender, mullein, myrrh, plantain, red sage, self-heal, St.-John's-wort, yarrow
Cystitis (see Urinary tract infection)		
Diarrhea	Goldenseal, licorice root, Oregon grape root, slippery elm	
Digestive problems (see Indigestion)		
Ear infection	Echinacea, goldenseal, oregano, Oregon grape root, thyme	Calendula, chamomile, clove oil, mullein, St.-John's-wort, witch hazel
Eczema and other inflammatory skin disorders	Burdock root, chickweed, cleavers, echinacea, goldenseal, nettle, Oregon grape root, red clover, sarsaparilla, yellow dock	Calendula, comfrey, lavender, nettle, yarrow
Epilepsy (see Seizures)		
Fever	Diaphoretics: catnip, cayenne, elder, ginger, peppermint, thyme, yarrow (*Note:* Since most fevers accompany an infection, see also Bacterial or viral infection)	
Flatulence (see Gas)		
Fungal infection		Arborvitae, calendula, echinacea, garlic, goldenseal
Gas	Aniseed, caraway, cardamom, catnip, cayenne, chamomile, cinnamon, clove, coriander, fennel, ginger, parsley, peppermint, thyme, valerian	
Gastritis	Chamomile, goldenseal, licorice, marsh mallow, slippery elm	

CONDITION	INTERNAL HERBS	EXTERNAL HERBS
Hepatitis	Artichoke, dandelion root, milk thistle, turmeric (*Note:* Also include herbs for bacterial infection)	
Hypothyroidism	Licorice, seaweed, Siberian ginseng	
Impotence	Damiana, ginkgo, *Panax ginseng,* saw palmetto	
Incontinence (see also Urinary tract infection)	Agrimony, horsetail	
Indigestion (dyspepsia)	Cardamom, catnip, cayenne, chamomile, cinnamon, clove, dandelion root, dill, fennel, ginger, peppermint, red sage, rosemary, thyme, valerian, wild yam	
Infection	Cayenne, cleavers, echinacea, garlic, ginger, goldenseal, lavender, myrrh, Oregon grape root, thyme	Echinacea, garlic, goldenseal, lavender, myrrh, Oregon grape root, thyme
Irritable bowel syndrome (see Colitis)		
Itching	Burdock root, calendula, chamomile, chickweed, cleavers, goldenseal, licorice root, Oregon grape root, sarsaparilla, St.-John's-wort, wild yam	Calendula, chamomile, echinacea, goldenseal, lavender, mullein, Oregon grape root, St.-John's-wort
Jaundice (see Hepatitis)		
Kidney disease	Cranberry (unsweetened juice), dandelion root, goldenseal, horsetail, marsh mallow root, Oregon grape root, parsley, Siberian ginseng, uva-ursi	
Kidney stones (see Urinary tract infection)		
Liver disease (see Hepatitis)		
Lyme disease and other tickborne diseases	Cat's claw, garlic, goldenseal, oregano, Oregon grape root	
Motion sickness	Ginger	

CONDITION	INTERNAL HERBS	EXTERNAL HERBS
Muscle sprains, strains, and pain	Arnica (homeopathic remedy only), cayenne, kava kava, licorice root, St.-John's-wort, turmeric, wild yam, willow bark	Arnica
Nephritis (see Kidney disease)		
Osteoarthritis (see Arthritis)		
Pain (general)	Black cohosh, black willow, cayenne, chamomile, hop, Jamaican dogwood, kava kava, licorice root, rosemary, St-John's-wort, skullcap, turmeric, valerian, wild lettuce, wild yam	Arnica, chamomile, echinacea, mullein
Pancreatitis	Dandelion root, goldenseal, licorice root, slippery elm	
Pink eye (see Conjunctivitis)		
Prostate disorders	Damiana, goldenseal, horsetail, nettle, Oregon grape root, oregano, pygeum, saw palmetto	
Psoriasis	Burdock, cleavers, flaxseed, licorice root, milk thistle, Oregon grape root, red clover, sarsaparilla, yellow dock	
Rheumatism (see Arthritis)		
Ringworm (see Fungal infection)		
Seizures	Chamomile, ginkgo, kava kava, licorice root, milk thistle, passionflower, St.-John's-wort, skullcap, valerian	
Sinusitis (see Upper respiratory disease)		
Stomach upset (see Indigestion)		
Ulcers	Goldenseal, licorice root, marsh mallow, Oregon grape root, slippery elm	
Ulcerative colitis (see Colitis)		

CONDITION	INTERNAL HERBS	EXTERNAL HERBS
Upper respiratory disease	Chamomile, echinacea, elder, eyebright, garlic, goldenseal, mullein, myrrh, Oregon grape root, oregano, peppermint, rose hip, thyme, yarrow	
Urinary tract infection	Cranberry (unsweetened juice), dandelion root, goldenseal, nettle, marsh mallow root, Oregon grape root, parsley, plantain, uva-ursi	
Viral infections (see Bacterial or viral infections)		
Vomiting	Cinnamon, clove, marsh mallow, meadowsweet, peppermint, rosemary, slippery elm	
Wart	Arborvitae (herbal and homeopathic)	Banana peel, arborvitae (herbal and homeopathic)
Wounds (see Cuts and scrapes)		
Yeast infections (see Fungal infections)		

Resources

For information on holistic veterinarians in your area, contact the American Holistic Veterinary Medicine Association. The Association's Web site lists holistic veterinarians by state and specifies the types of alternative medicine that each vet uses.

American Holistic Veterinary Medicine Association
410-569-0795
www.ahvma.org

SUGGESTED READING

General Holistic Health Care Books for Pets

Frazier, Anitra. *The New Natural Cat.* Dutton, 1990.

Levy, Juliette de Bairacli. *Cats Naturally.* Faber and Faber, 1991.

Levy, Juliette de Bairacli. *The Complete Herbal Handbook for the Dog and Cat.* Faber and Faber, 1995.

Pitcairn, Richard. *Dr. Pitcairn's Complete Guide to Natural Health for Dogs and Cats.* Rodale, 1995.

General Herbal Books

Buhner, Stephen Harrod. *Herbal Antibiotics.* Storey Publishing, 1999.

Duke, James A. *The Green Pharmacy.* Rodale, 1997.

Foster, Steven. *Herbal Renaissance.* Gibbs Smith, 1993.

Foster, Steven and Varro E. Tyler. *Tyler's Honest Herbal.* Hawthorn Herbal Press, 1999.

Gladstar, Rosemary. *Herbal Healing for Women.* Fireside, 1993.

Gladstar, Rosemary. *Rosemary Gladstar's Herbal Remedies for Children's Health.* Storey Publishing, 1999.

Hoffman, David. *The New Holistic Herbal.* Element, 1991.

Mowery, Daniel B. *Herbal Tonic Therapies.* Random House, 1996.

Murray, Michael. *The Healing Power of Herbs.* Prima Publishing, 1995.

Tierra, Michael. *Way of Herbs.* Pocket Books, 1998.

Wood, Matthew. *The Book of Herbal Wisdom.* North Atlantic Books, 1997.

Magazines

The Essential Herbal
www.essentialherbal.com

The Herb Companion
800-456-5835
www.herbcompanion.com

The Herb Quarterly
510-668-0268
www.herbquarterly.com

The Herbal Collective Magazine
250-722-7108
www.herbalcollective.ca

Herbs for Health
800-456-6018
www.herbsforhealth.com

HerbalGram
512-926-4900
www.herbalgram.org

Journal of Herbs, Spices & Medicinal Plants
www.tandf.co.uk/journals/WHSM

The Whole Dog Journal
800-829-9165
www.whole-dog-journal.com
An excellent holistic newsletter with occasional herbal information.

Index

Note: Page number in *italic* refer to illustrations; those in **boldface** refer to charts.

Other Storey Titles You Will Enjoy

The Cat Behavior Answer Book, by Arden Moore.
Practical insights into the feline mind — for cat
owners everywhere!
336 pages. Flexibind. ISBN 978-1-58017-674-3.

Dr. Kidd's Guide to Herbal Cat Care, by Randy Kidd, DVM, PhD.
Thorough information on using all-natural herbal remedies to
treat and prevent disease in your favorite feline.
208 pages. Paper. ISBN 978-1-58017-188-5.

The Dog Behavior Answer Book, by Arden Moore.
Answers to your questions about canine quirks,
baffling habits, and destructive behavior.
336 pages. Flexibind. ISBN 978-1-58017-644-6.

Happy Dog, Happy You, by Arden Moore.
Gentle humor and inspired advice from a pet expert
to owners and their canine friends.
304 pages. Paper. ISBN 978-1-60342-032-7.

The Puppy Owner's Manual, by Diana Delmar.
How to solve all your puppy problems and create
a puppy-friendly home.
192 pages. Paper. ISBN 978-1-58017-401-5.

Real Food for Dogs, by Arden Moore.
A collection of 50 vet-approved recipes to please
your canine gastronome.
128 pages. Paper. ISBN 978-1-58017-424-4.

These and other books from Storey Publishing are available
wherever quality books are sold or by calling 1-800-441-5700.
Visit us at *www.storey.com.*